WHY WE LOVE DOGS,
EAT PIGS, AND WEAR COWS

WHY WE
LOVE DOGS

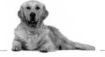

EAT PIGS

AND
WEAR COWS

An INTRODUCTION *to* **CARNISM**

The Belief System That Enables Us to Eat Some Animals and Not Others

Melanie Joy, Ph.D.

Conari Press

First published in 2010 by Conari Press,
an imprint of Red Wheel/Weiser, LLC
With offices at:
500 Third Street, Suite 230
San Francisco, CA 94107
www.redwheelweiser.com

ISBN: 978-1-57324-461-9
Library of Congress Cataloging-in-Publication Data is available upon request.

Cover design by Stewart A. Williams
Text design by Donna Linden
Typeset in Clarendon, Excelsior, and Perpetua
Cover photographs: dog © Eric Isselée/iStockphoto.com; bacon © Arpad
Benedek/iStockphoto.com; shoes © Andrew Johnson/iStockphoto.com

Printed in the United States of America
MV
10 9 8 7 6 5 4 3 2

The paper used in this publication meets the minimum requirements of the American National Standard for Information Sciences—Permanence of Paper for Printed
Library Materials Z39.48-1992 (R1997).

For witnesses everywhere.
Through your eyes, we may find our way.

The greatness of a nation and its moral progress can be judged by the way its animals are treated.
—Mahatma Gandhi

CONTENTS

ACKNOWLEDGMENTS

This book is the result of a project that began many years ago, with an idea that turned into a doctoral dissertation, which then grew into the volume it is today. Over the years, many people helped shape my ideas and hone my words, and supported me as a professional and a person. To them I am eternally grateful. I want to thank Aimee Houser, my brilliant and inspiring editor, who worked with me every step of the way; my agent, Patti Breitman, who believed in my work and made sure it found a home; Erik Williams, my partner and friend, whose love sustains me; Clare Seletsky, who carried this project through the home stretch; Caroline Pincus and Bonni Hamilton of Red Wheel/Weiser, for their enthusiasm and support; Carolyn Zaikowski, who insisted that I write this book; Bonnie Tardella, for her tireless editing; Janice Goldman, George Bournakis, Herb Pearce, and Susan Solomon for being my lifelines; Anna Meigs, for her wisdom and guidance; Ruth and Jake Tedaldi, for helping me when I most needed it; Teri Jessen, for her vision; Bonnie and Perry Norton, for believing in me and giving me the opportunity to carry out my work; Fred and Claudette Williams; Dina Aronson; John Adams; Stephen Cina; Adam Wake; Linda Riebel; Michael Greger; Zoe Weil; V. K. Kool; Ken Shapiro; Stephen Shainbart; Hillary Rettig; Rita Agrawal; Eric Prescott; Laureano Batista; Josh Balk; and Robin Stone. I also want to thank my friends and family who have supported me throughout a very long journey.

CHAPTER 1

TO LOVE OR TO EAT?

We don't see things as they are; we see them as we are.
—Anais Nin

Imagine, for a moment, the following scenario: You are a guest at an elegant dinner party. You're seated with the other guests at an ornately set table. The room is warm, candlelight flickers across crystal wineglasses, and the conversation is flowing freely. Mouthwatering smells of rich foods emanate from the kitchen. You haven't eaten all day, and your stomach is growling.

At last, after what feels like hours, your friend who is hosting the party emerges from the kitchen with a steaming pot of savory stew. The aromas of meat, seasonings, and vegetables fill the room. You serve yourself a generous portion, and after eating several mouthfuls of tender meat, you ask your friend for the recipe.

"I'd be happy to tell you," she replies. "You begin with five pounds of golden retriever meat, well marinated, and then . . ." *Golden retriever?* You probably freeze midbite as you consider her words: the meat in your mouth is from a *dog.*

What now? Do you continue eating? Or are you revolted by the fact that there's golden retriever on your plate, and you've just eaten some? Do you pick out the meat and eat the vegetables around it? If you are like most Americans, when you hear that you've been eating dog, your feelings would automatically change from pleasure to some degree of revulsion.* You might also become turned off by the vegetables in the stew, as if they were somehow tainted by the meat.

But let's suppose that your friend laughs and says she was playing a practical joke. The meat isn't golden retriever, after all, but beef. How do you feel about your food now? Is your appetite fully restored? Do you resume eating with the same enthusiasm you had when you first began your meal? Chances are, even though you know that the stew on your plate is exactly the same food you were savoring just moments earlier, you would have some residual emotional discomfort, discomfort that might continue to affect you the next time you sit down to beef stew.

What's going on here? Why is it that certain foods cause such emotional reactions? How can a food, given one label, be considered highly palatable and that same food, given another, become virtually inedible? The stew's main ingredient—meat—didn't really change at all. It was animal flesh to begin with, and it remained that way. It just became— or seemed to, for a moment—meat from a different animal. Why is it that we have such radically different reactions to beef and dog meat?

The answer to these questions can be summed up by a single word: *perception*. We react differently to different types of meat not because there is a physical difference between them, but because our perception of them is different.

The Problem with Eating Dogs

Such a shift in perception can feel like a shift in lanes on a two-lane road: crossing the yellow line radically alters our experience. The reason we can have such a powerful response to a shift in perception

---

*Although some individuals might be intrigued rather than repulsed at the idea of eating dogs, in the United States these people represent a minority, and this book describes the experience of Americans in general.

is because our perceptions determine, in large part, our reality; how we perceive a situation—the meaning we make of it—determines what we think and how we feel about it. In turn, our thoughts and feelings often determine how we will act. Most Americans perceive dog meat very differently than they do beef; therefore, dog meat evokes very different mental, emotional, and behavioral responses.[*]

One reason we have such different perceptions of beef and dog meat is because we view cows[**] and dogs very differently. The most frequent—and often the only—contact we have with cows is when we eat (or wear) them. But for a large number of Americans, our relationship with dogs is, in many ways, not terribly different from our relationship with people: We call them by their names. We say goodbye when we leave and greet them when we return. We share our beds with them. We play with them. We buy them gifts. We carry their pictures in our wallets. We take them to the doctor when they're sick and may spend thousands of dollars on their treatment. We bury them when they pass away. They make us laugh; they make us cry. They are our helpers, our friends, our family. We love them. We love dogs and eat cows not because dogs and cows are fundamentally different—cows, like dogs, have feelings, preferences, and consciousness—but because our *perception* of them is different. And, consequently, our perception of their meat is different as well.

---

[*]In cultures around the world, it is common to reject the meat of certain animal species. And taboos regarding the consumption of meat are far more common than those regarding any other foods. Moreover, violations of meat taboos cause the strongest emotional reactions—generally, disgust—and are accompanied by the most severe sanctions. Consider the dietary prohibitions put forth by the major religions of the world; whether the restriction is temporary (as when Christians avoid meat during Lent) or permanent (as with some Buddhists who maintain a vegetarian lifestyle), meat is almost always the object of the taboo.

[**]Though beef comes from both cows and steers, for simplicity and style I use "cows" throughout this chapter to refer to all bovines.

ot only do our perceptions of meat vary based on the species
nal it came from, but different humans may also perceive the
same meat differently. For example, a Hindu might have the same
response to beef as an American Christian would to dog meat. These
variations in our perceptions are due to our *schema*. A schema is a psychological framework that shapes—and is shaped by—our beliefs,
ideas, perceptions, and experiences, and it automatically organizes and
interprets incoming information. For example, when you hear the word
"nurse," you probably envision a woman who wears a medical uniform
and works in a hospital. Even though a number of nurses are male, dress
nontraditionally, or work outside of a hospital, unless you are frequently
exposed to nurses in a variety of settings, your schema will maintain this
generalized image. Generalizations are the result of schemas doing what
they're supposed to: sorting through and interpreting the vast amount
of stimuli we're constantly exposed to and then putting it into general
categories. Schemas act as mental classification systems.

We have a schema for every subject, including animals. An animal
can be classified, for instance, as prey, predator, pest, pet, or food. How
we classify an animal, in turn, determines how we relate to it*—whether
we hunt it, flee from it, exterminate it, love it, or eat it. Some overlap
can occur between categories (an animal can be prey *and* food), but when
it comes to meat, most animals are either food, or not food. In other
words, we have a schema that classifies animals as edible or inedible.**

------

*I realize that some readers may be uncomfortable with my use of language in reference
to nonhuman animals. I have chosen to use speciesist terms such as "it" simply to keep the
text colloquial and to avoid distracting readers from its content.
**Schemas can be hierarchically structured, with sub-schemas embedded in more com-
plex or general schemas. For example, we have a general schema for "animal" and within
this are sub-schemas of "edible" and "inedible." These sub-schemas, in turn, can be broken
down into further sub-schemas; for instance "edible" animals may consist of "wild game,"
and "domesticated" or "farm" animals.

And something interesting happens when we are confronted with the meat from an animal we've classified as inedible: we automatically picture the living animal from which it came, and we tend to feel disgusted at the notion of eating it. The perceptual process follows this sequence:

golden retriever meat (stimulus) ⟶ *inedible animal (belief/perception)* ⟶ *image of living dog (thought)* ⟶ *disgust (feeling)* ⟶ *refusal or reluctance to eat (action)*

Let's go back to our imagined dinner party, when you were told you were eating golden retriever. Had such a situation actually occurred, you would have smelled the same smells and tasted the same flavors as you had just moments before. But now your mind probably would have formed a picture of a golden retriever, perhaps bounding across a yard chasing a ball, curled up next to a fire, or running alongside a jogger. And with these images would likely come emotions such as empathy or concern for the dog that had been killed and thus disgust at the thought of eating that animal.

In contrast, if you are like most people, when you sit down to eat beef you don't envision the animal from which the meat was derived. Instead, you simply see "food," and you focus on its flavor, aroma, and texture. When confronted with beef, we generally skip the part of the perceptual process that makes the mental connection between meat and the living animal. Sure, we all know that beef comes from an animal, but when we eat it, we tend to avoid thinking about this fact. Literally thousands of people with whom I have spoken, both through my professional work and personally, have admitted that if they actually thought about a living cow while eating beef they would feel uneasy—and sometimes even unable to eat it. This is why many people avoid eating meat that resembles the animal from which it was procured; rarely is our meat served with the head or other body parts intact. In one interesting study, for instance, Danish researchers found that people were uncomfortable eating meat that resembled its animal source, preferring to eat minced meat rather than whole cuts of meat.[1] Yet even if we do make the conscious connection between beef and cows, we still feel less disturbed eating beef than we would eating golden retriever, since typically in American culture, dogs are not meant to be eaten.

How we feel about an animal and how we treat it, it turns out, has much less to do with what kind of animal it is than about what our perception of it is. We believe it's appropriate to eat cows but not dogs, so we perceive cows as edible and dogs as inedible and act accordingly. And this process is cyclical; not only do our beliefs ultimately lead to our actions, but our actions also reinforce our beliefs. The more we don't eat dogs and do eat cows, the more we reinforce the belief that dogs are inedible and cows are edible.

Acquired Taste

While human beings may have an innate tendency to favor sweet flavors (sugar having been a useful source of calories) and to avoid those that are bitter and sour (such flavors often indicate a poisonous substance), most of our taste is, in fact, made up. In other words, within the broad repertoire of the human palate, we like the foods we've learned we're *supposed* to like. Food, particularly animal food, is highly symbolic, and it is this symbolism, coupled with and reinforced by tradition, that is largely responsible for our food preferences. For example, few people enjoy eating caviar until they're old enough to realize that liking caviar means they're sophisticated and refined; and in China, people eat animals' penises because they believe these organs affect sexual function.

Despite the fact that taste is largely acquired through culture, people around the world tend to view their preferences as rational and any deviation as offensive and disgusting. For instance, many people are disgusted at the thought of drinking milk that's been extracted from cows' udders. Others cannot fathom eating bacon, ham, beef, or chicken. Some view the consumption of eggs as akin to the consumption of fetuses (which, technically, it is). And consider how you might feel at the notion of eating deep-fried tarantula (hair, fangs, and all), as they do in Cambodia; sour, pickled ram's testicle pâté, as some do in Iceland; or duck embryos—eggs that have been fertilized and contain partially formed birds with feathers, bones, and incipient wings—as they do in some parts of Asia. When it comes to animal foods, all taste may be acquired taste.[2]

The Missing Link

It is an odd phenomenon, the way we react to the idea of eating dogs and other inedible animals. Even stranger, though, is the way we *don't* react to the idea of eating cows and other edible animals. There is an unexplained gap, a missing link, in our perceptual process when it comes to edible species; we fail to make the connection between meat and its animal source. Have you ever wondered why, out of tens of thousands of animal species, you probably feel disgusted at the idea of eating all but a tiny handful of them? What is most striking about our selection of edible and inedible animals is not the *presence* of disgust, but the *absence* of it. Why are we *not* averse to eating the very small selection of animals we have deemed edible?[3]

The evidence strongly suggests that our lack of disgust is largely, if not entirely, learned. We aren't born with our schemas; they are constructed. Our schemas have evolved out of a highly structured belief system. This system dictates which animals are edible, and it enables us to consume them by protecting us from feeling any emotional or psychological discomfort when doing so. The system teaches us how to *not feel*. The most obvious feeling we lose is disgust, yet beneath our disgust lies an emotion much more integral to our sense of self: our empathy.

From Empathy to Apathy

But why must the system go to such lengths to block our empathy? Why all the psychological acrobatics? The answer is simple: because we care about animals, and we don't want them to suffer. And because we eat them. Our values and behaviors are incongruent, and this incongruence causes us a certain degree of moral discomfort. In order to alleviate this discomfort, we have three choices: we can change our values to match our behaviors, we can change our behaviors to match our values, or we can change our *perception* of our behaviors so that they *appear* to match our values. It is around this third option that our schema of meat is shaped. As long as we neither value unnecessary animal suffering nor stop eating animals, our schema will distort our perceptions of animals and the meat we eat, so that we can feel comfortable enough to consume them. And the system that constructs our schema of meat equips us with the means by which to do this.

The primary tool of the system is *psychic numbing*. Psychic numbing is a psychological process by which we disconnect, mentally and emotionally, from our experience; we "numb" ourselves. In and of itself, psychic numbing is not evil; it is a normal, inevitable part of daily life, enabling us to function in a violent and unpredictable world and to cope with our pain if we do fall prey to violence. For instance, you would likely be hard-pressed to drive on the highway if you were fully cognizant of the fact that you were speeding down the road in a small metal vehicle, surrounded by thousands of other speeding metal vehicles. And if you should be so unfortunate as to become a victim of a crash, you would probably go into shock and remain in that state until you were psychologically capable of handling the reality of what had happened. Psychic numbing is adaptive, or beneficial, when it helps us to *cope* with violence. But it becomes maladaptive, or destructive, when it is used to *enable* violence, even if that violence is as far away as the factories in which animals are turned into meat.

Psychic numbing is made up of a complex array of defenses and other mechanisms, mechanisms which are pervasive, powerful, and invisible and which operate on both social and psychological levels. These mechanisms distort our perceptions and distance us from our feelings, transforming our empathy into apathy—indeed, it is the process of learning to not feel that is the focus of this book. The mechanisms of psychic numbing include: denial, avoidance, routinization, justification, objectification, deindividualization, dichotomization, rationalization, and dissociation. In the upcoming chapters, we will examine each of these aspects of psychic numbing and deconstruct the system that turns animals into meat, and meat into food. In so doing, we will examine the characteristics of this system and the ways in which it ensures our continued support.

Numbing Across Cultures and History: Variations on a Theme

One question I'm often asked is whether people from different cultures and times also have used psychic numbing in order to kill and consume animals. Do tribal huntsmen, for instance, need to numb themselves when securing their prey? Before the Industrial Revolution, when many Americans procured their own meat, did they have to emotionally distance themselves from the animals?

It would be impossible to argue that persons from all cultures, in all eras, have employed the same psychic numbing as those of us living in contemporary industrialized societies and who don't need meat to survive. Context determines, in large part, how a person will react to eating meat. One's values, shaped largely by broader social and cultural structures, help determine how much psychological effort must go into distancing oneself from the reality of eating an animal. In societies where meat has been necessary for survival, people haven't had the luxury of reflecting on the ethics of their choices; their values must support eating animals, and they would likely be less distressed at the notion of eating meat. How animals are killed, too, affects our psychological reaction. Cruelty is often more disturbing than killing.

Yet even in instances where eating meat has been a necessity, and the animals have been killed without the gratuitous violence that marks today's slaughterhouses, people have always avoided eating certain types of animals and have consistently striven to reconcile the killing and consumption of those they do consume. Examples abound of rites, rituals, and belief systems that assuage the meat consumer's conscience: the butcher and/or meat eater may perform purification ceremonies after the taking of a life; or an animal may be viewed as "sacrificed" for human consumption, a perspective that imbues the act with spiritual meaning and implies some choice on the part of the prey. Furthermore, as far back as 600 BCE, individuals have chosen to eschew the consumption of meat on ethical grounds, demonstrating a long-standing psychological and moral tension around meat eating. It is certainly possible that psychic numbing has played a role—albeit to varying degrees and in different forms—across cultures and throughout history.

The primary defense of the system is invisibility; invisibility reflects the defenses *avoidance* and *denial* and is the foundation on which all other mechanisms stand. Invisibility enables us, for example, to consume beef without envisioning the animal we're eating; it cloaks our thoughts from ourselves. Invisibility also keeps us safely insulated from the unpleasant process of raising and killing animals for our food. The first step in deconstructing meat, then, is deconstructing the invisibility of the system, exposing the principles and practices of a system that has since its inception been in hiding.

CHAPTER 2

CARNISM:

"IT'S JUST THE WAY THINGS ARE"

The invisible and the nonexistent look very much alike.
—*Delos B. McKown*

The limits of my language mean the limits of my world.
—*Ludwig Wittgenstein*

In chapter 1, we did a thought experiment. We imagined that you were at a dinner party, eating a delicious meal, when your friend told you the stew contained dog meat. We explored your reactions to that, and then to the fact that your friend said she'd been joking and you were, in fact, eating beef.

Let's try another exercise. Take a moment to think, without self-censoring, of all the words that come to mind when you envision a dog. Next, do the same thing, but this time picture a pig. Now pause and compare your descriptions of these animals. What do you notice? When you thought of a dog, did you think "cute"? "Loyal"? And when you imagined a pig, did you think of the word "mud" or "sweat"? Did you think "dirty"? If your responses were similar to the ones here, you are in the majority.

I teach psychology and sociology at a local university, and each semester I dedicate one class session to attitudes toward animals. I have taught literally thousands of students over the years, but every time we do this exercise, the conversation proceeds in essentially the same way, with similar responses.

First, as I just had you do, I ask the students to list the characteristics of dogs, and then the characteristics of pigs, and I write each list on the board as it's generated. For dogs, the usual adjectives include those we've already covered, as well as "friendly," "intelligent," "fun," "loving," "protective," and sometimes "dangerous." Not surprisingly, pigs get a much less flattering list of descriptives. They are "sweaty" and "dirty," as well as "stupid," "lazy," "fat," and "ugly." Next, I have the students explain how they feel toward each of these species. Again, it should come as no surprise that, generally, they at least like—and often love—dogs, and are "grossed out" by pigs. Finally, I ask them to describe their relationship to dogs and to pigs. Dogs, of course, are our friends and family members, and pigs are food.

At this point the students start to look perplexed, wondering where our conversation is heading. I then pose a series of questions in response to their previous statements, and the dialogue goes something like this:

So, why do you say pigs are lazy?
Because they just lie around all day.
Do pigs in the wild do this, or only pigs raised for their meat?
I don't know. Maybe when they're on a farm.
Why do you think pigs on a farm—or in a factory farm, to be
    more accurate—lie around?
Probably because they're in a pen or cage.

What makes pigs stupid?
They just are.
Actually, pigs are considered to be even more intelligent than
    dogs.

(Sometimes a student chimes in, claiming to have met a pig or to have known someone who had a pig as a pet, and corroborates this with a story or two.)

Why do you say pigs sweat?
No answer.
Did you know that, in fact, pigs don't even have sweat glands?

Are all pigs ugly?
Yes.
What about piglets?
Piglets are cute, but pigs are gross.

Why do you say pigs are dirty?
They roll in mud.
Why do they roll in mud?
Because they like dirt. They're dirty.
Actually, they roll in dirt to cool off when it's hot, since they don't sweat.

Are *dogs* dirty?
Yeah, sometimes. Dogs can do really disgusting things.
Why didn't you include "dirty" in your list for dogs?
Because they're not always dirty. Only sometimes.
Are pigs always dirty?
Yeah, they are.
How do you know this?
Because they always look dirty.
When do you see them?
I don't know. In pictures, I guess.
And they're always dirty in pictures?
No, not always. Pigs aren't always dirty.

You said dogs are loyal, intelligent, and cute. Why do you say this? How do you know?

I've seen them.

I've lived with dogs.

I've met lots of dogs.

(Inevitably, one or more students share a story about a dog who did something particularly heroic, clever, or adorable.)

What about dogs' feelings? How can you know that they actually feel emotions?

I swear my dog gets depressed when I'm down.

My dog always got this guilty look and hid under the bed when she knew she did something wrong.

Whenever we take my dog to the vet he shakes, he's so scared.

Our dog used to cry and stop eating when he saw us packing to get ready to leave for vacation.

Does anybody here think it's possible that dogs don't have feelings?

(No hands are raised.)

What about pigs? Do you think pigs have emotions?

Sure.

Do you think they have the same emotions as dogs?

Maybe. Yeah, I guess.

Actually, most people don't know this, but pigs are so sensitive that they develop neurotic behaviors, such as self-mutilation, when in captivity.

Do you think pigs feel pain?

Of course. All animals feel pain.

So why do we eat pigs and not dogs?

Because bacon tastes good (laughter).

Because dogs have personalities. You can't eat something that has a personality. They have names; they're individuals.

Do you think pigs have personalities? Are they individuals, like dogs?

Yeah, I guess if you get to know them they probably do.

Have you ever met a pig?

(Except for an exceptional student, the majority has not.)

So where did you get your information about pigs from?

Books.

Television.

Ads.

Movies.

I don't know. Society, I guess.

How might you feel about pigs if you thought of them as intelligent, sensitive individuals who are perhaps not sweaty, lazy, and greedy? If you got to know them firsthand, like you know dogs?

I'd feel weird eating them. I'd probably feel kind of guilty.

So why do we eat pigs and not dogs?

Because pigs are bred to be eaten.

Why do we breed pigs to eat them?

I don't know. I never thought about it. I guess, because it's just the way things are.

It's just the way things are. Take a moment to consider this statement. Really think about it. We send one species to the butcher and give our love and kindness to another apparently for no reason other than because *it's the way things are.* When our attitudes and behaviors toward animals are so inconsistent, and this inconsistency is so unexamined, we can safely say we have been fed absurdities. It is absurd that we eat pigs and love dogs and don't even know why. Many of us spend long minutes in the aisle of the drugstore mulling over what toothpaste to buy. Yet most of us don't spend any time at all thinking about what species of animal we eat and why. Our choices as consumers drive an industry that kills ten billion* animals per year in the United States alone. If we choose to support this industry and the best reason we can come up with is because it's the way things are, clearly something is amiss. What could cause an entire society of people to check their thinking caps at the door—*and to not even realize they're doing so?* Though this question is quite complex, the answer is quite simple: carnism.

Carnism

We all know what a vegetarian is—a person who doesn't eat meat. Though some people may choose to become vegetarian to improve their health, many vegetarians stop eating meat because they don't believe it's ethical to eat animals. Most of us realize that vegetarianism is an expression of one's ethical orientation, so when we think of a vegetarian, we don't simply think of a person who's just like everyone else except that he or she doesn't eat meat. We think of a person who has a certain philosophical outlook, whose choice not to eat meat is a reflection of a deeper belief system in which killing animals for human ends is considered unethical. We understand that vegetarianism reflects not merely a dietary orientation, but a way of life. This is why, for instance, when there's a vegetarian character in a movie, he or she is depicted not simply as a person who avoids meat,

---

*Though billions of sea creatures are also slaughtered annually in the United States, unless otherwise noted, the "food" animals I refer to are land animals.

but as someone who has a certain set of qualities that we associate with vegetarians, such as being a nature lover or having unconventional values.

If a vegetarian is someone who believes that it's unethical to eat meat, what, then, do we call a person who believes that it's ethical to eat meat? If a vegetarian is a person who chooses not to eat meat, what is a person who chooses *to* eat meat?

Currently, we use the term "meat eater" to describe anyone who is not vegetarian. But how accurate is this? As we established, a vegetarian is not simply a "plant eater." Eating plants is a *behavior* that stems from a belief system. "Vegetarian" accurately reflects that a core belief system is at work: the suffix "arian" denotes a person who advocates, supports, or practices a doctrine or set of principles.

In contrast, the term "meat eater" isolates the practice of consuming meat, as though it were divorced from a person's beliefs and values. It implies that the person who eats meat is acting *outside* of a belief system. But is eating meat truly a behavior that exists independent of a belief system? Do we eat pigs and not dogs because we don't have a belief system when it comes to eating animals?

In much of the industrialized world, we eat meat not because we have to; we eat meat because we choose to. We don't need meat to survive or even to be healthy; millions of healthy and long-lived vegetarians have proven this point. We eat animals simply because it's what we've always done, and because we like the way they taste. Most of us eat animals because it's just the way things are.

We don't see meat eating as we do vegetarianism—as a choice, based on a set of assumptions about animals, our world, and ourselves. Rather, we see it as a given, the "natural" thing to do, the way things have always been and the way things will always be. We eat animals without thinking about what we are doing and why because the belief system that underlies this behavior is invisible. This invisible belief system is what I call *carnism*.

Carnism is the belief system in which eating certain animals is considered ethical and appropriate. Carnists—people who eat meat—are not the same as carnivores. Carnivores are animals that are dependent on meat to survive. Carnists are also not merely omnivores. An omnivore is an animal—human or nonhuman—that has the physiological ability to ingest both plants and meat. But, like "carnivore," "omnivore" is a term that describes one's biological constitution, not one's philosophical choice. Carnists eat meat not because they need to, but because they choose to, and choices always stem from beliefs.

Carnism's invisibility accounts for why choices appear not to be choices at all. But why has carnism remained invisible in the first place? Why haven't we named it? There's a very good reason for this. It's because carnism is a particular type of belief system, an *ideology,* and it's also a particular type of ideology, one that is especially resistant to scrutiny. Let's look at each of these features of carnism in turn.

> *If the problem is invisible . . .*
> *then there will be ethical invisibility.*
> *—Carol J. Adams*

Carnism, Ideology, and the Status Quo

An ideology is a shared set of beliefs, as well as the practices that reflect these beliefs. For instance, feminism is an ideology. Feminists are men and women who believe that women deserve to be viewed and treated as equals to men. Because men make up the dominant social group—the group that holds power in society—feminists challenge male dominance on every front, from the home to the political arena. Feminist ideology forms the basis of feminist beliefs and practices.

It's fairly easy to recognize feminism as an ideology, just as it's easy to understand that vegetarianism isn't simply about not eating meat.

Both "feminist" and "vegetarian" conjure up images of a person who has a certain set of beliefs, someone who isn't just like everybody else.

So what about "everybody else"? What about the majority, the mainstream, all the "normal" people? Where do their beliefs come from?

We tend to view the mainstream way of life as a reflection of universal values. Yet what we consider normal is, in fact, nothing more than the beliefs and behaviors of the majority. Before the scientific revolution, for example, mainstream European beliefs held that the sky was made up of heavenly spheres that revolved around the earth, that the earth was the exalted center of the universe. This belief was so ingrained that to proclaim otherwise, as did Copernicus, and later Galileo, was to risk death. So what we refer to as mainstream is simply another way to describe an ideology that is so widespread—so *entrenched*—that its assumptions and practices are seen as simply common sense. It is considered fact rather than opinion, its practices a given rather than a choice. It's the norm. It's the way things are. And it's the reason carnism has not been named until now.

When an ideology is entrenched, it is essentially invisible. An example of an invisible ideology is *patriarchy*, the ideology in which masculinity is valued over femininity and where men therefore have more social power than women. Consider, for instance, which of the following qualities are most likely to make someone socially and financially successful: assertiveness, passivity, competitiveness, sharing, control, authority, power, rationality, emotionality, independence, dependence, nurturance, vulnerability. Chances are you chose the qualities that are masculine, and you didn't realize that your choices reflect patriarchal values; most of us don't see patriarchy as an ideology that teaches us to think and act a certain way. Men and women alike simply accept that it's better to be, for example, more rational and less emotional, even though both of these qualities are equally necessary for our well-being.

Patriarchy existed for thousands of years before feminists named this ideology. So, too, has been the case with carnism. Interestingly, the ideology of vegetarianism was named more than 2,500 years ago; those who chose not to eat meat were called "Pythagoreans," because they followed the dietary philosophy of the ancient Greek philosopher and mathematician, Pythagoras. Later, in the nineteenth century, the term "vegetarian" was coined. But only now, centuries after labeling those who don't eat meat, has the ideology of meat eating been named.

In some ways it only makes sense that vegetarianism was named before carnism. It's easier to recognize those ideologies that fall outside the mainstream. But there is another, more important, reason that vegetarianism has been labeled while carnism has not. The primary way entrenched ideologies stay entrenched is by remaining invisible. And the primary way they stay invisible is by remaining unnamed. If we don't name it, we can't talk about it, and if we can't talk about it, we can't question it.

> *Whatever is unnamed, undepicted in images . . . whatever is misnamed as something else, made difficult-to-come-by, whatever is buried in the memory by the collapse of meaning under an inadequate or lying language— this will become, not merely unspoken, but unspeakable.*
> *—Adrienne Rich*

Carnism, Ideology, and Violence

While it is difficult, if not impossible, to question an ideology that we don't even know exists, it's even more difficult when that ideology actively works to keep itself hidden. This is the case with ideologies such as carnism. I refer to this particular type of ideology as a *violent ideology,* because it is literally organized around physical violence. In other words, if we were to remove the violence from the system—to stop killing animals—the system would cease to exist. Meat cannot be procured without slaughter.

Contemporary carnism is organized around extensive violence. This level of violence is necessary in order to slaughter enough animals for the meat industry to maintain its current profit margin. The violence of carnism is such that most people are unwilling to witness it, and those who do can become seriously distraught. In my classes, when I show a film on meat production, I have to take a number of measures to ensure that the psychological environment is safe enough to expose students to footage that inevitably causes them distress. And I have personally worked with numerous vegetarian advocates who suffer from post-traumatic stress disorder (PTSD) as the result of prolonged exposure to the slaughter process; they have intrusive thoughts, nightmares, flashbacks, difficulty concentrating, anxiety, insomnia, and a host of other symptoms. In close to two decades of speaking and teaching about meat production, I have yet to see a person who doesn't cringe when faced with images of slaughter. People generally hate to see animals suffer.

Why do we hate to see animals in pain? Because we feel for other sentient beings. Most of us, even those who are not "animal lovers" per se, don't want to cause anyone—human or animal—to suffer, especially if that suffering is intensive and unnecessary. It is for this reason that violent ideologies have a special set of defenses that enable humane people to support inhumane practices and to not even realize what they're doing.

Unnatural Born Killers

There is a substantial body of evidence demonstrating humans' seemingly natural aversion to killing. Much of the research in this area has been conducted by the military; analysts have found that soldiers tend to intentionally fire over the enemy's head, or not to fire at all.

Studies of combat activity during the Napoleonic and Civil Wars revealed striking statistics. Given the ability of the men, their proximity to the enemy, and the capacity of their weapons, the number of enemy soldiers hit should have been well over 50 percent, resulting in a killing rate of hundreds per minute. Instead, however, the hit rate was only one or two per minute. And a similar phenomenon occurred during World War I: according to British lieutenant George Roupell, the only way he could get his men to stop firing into the air was by drawing his sword, walking down the trench, "beating [them] on the backside and . . . telling them to fire low."[4] World War II fire rates were also remarkably low: historian and U.S. Army brigadier general S. L. A. Marshall reported that, during battle, the firing rate was a mere 15 to 20 percent; in other words, out of every hundred men engaged in a firefight, only fifteen to twenty actually used their weapons. And in Vietnam, for every enemy soldier killed, more than fifty thousand bullets were fired.[5]

What these studies have taught the military is that in order to get soldiers to shoot to kill, to actively participate in violence, the soldiers must be sufficiently desensitized to the act of killing. In other words, they have to *learn to not feel*—

and to not feel responsible—for their actions. They must be taught to override their own conscience. Yet these studies also demonstrate that even in the face of immediate danger, in situations of extreme violence, most people are averse to killing. In other words, as Marshall concludes, "the vast majority of combatants throughout history, at the moment of truth when they could and should kill the enemy, have found themselves to be 'conscientious objectors.'"[6]

As I mentioned in chapter 1, the primary defense of the system is invisibility. We've already discussed how carnism is socially and psychologically invisible. But violent ideologies also depend on physical invisibility; their violence is well hidden from public scrutiny. Have you ever noticed that, though we breed, raise, and kill ten billion animals per year, most of us never see even a single part of the process of meat production?

Once we genuinely think about the meat we eat, once we realize that there is much more to our culinary tastes than our own natural, unadulterated preferences, then "it's just the way things are" is simply not a good enough explanation for why we eat pigs but not dogs. Let's turn now and have a look at the way things really are.

CHAPTER 3

THE WAY THINGS *REALLY* ARE

Make the lie big, make it simple, keep saying it,
and eventually they will believe it.
—Adolf Hitler

If you are like most Americans, meat is a staple of your diet. You probably eat meat at least once a day, if not more often. Think about the foods you've eaten over the past week. How many meals have you had that consisted of some form of chicken, beef, pork, or turkey? Have you had bacon or sausage with your breakfast? Roast beef or turkey sandwiches for lunch? Rotisserie or fried chicken for dinner? How much meat do you think you've eaten this week? This month? This year?

The U.S. Department of Agriculture (USDA) estimates that the average American consumes 87 pounds of chicken, 17 pounds of turkey, 66 pounds of beef, and 51 pounds of pork per year. Add to this a pound of veal and a pound of lamb, and each of us eats a total of 223 pounds of meat annually.[7] Given that the current population of the United States is 300 million, that's a lot of meat—and a lot of animals.

To be exact, U.S. agribusinesses slaughter *ten billion* animals per year, and that's not including the estimated ten billion fish and other sea animals that are killed annually. That's 19,011 animals per minute, or 317 animals per second. In the time it took you to read these three paragraphs, nearly 60,000 more animals were killed.

Just to give you some perspective, the ten billion U.S. farm-animal population is nearly double the size of the worldwide human population. It's 33 times larger than the population of the United States, 1,250 times higher than the population of New York City, and 2,500 times larger than the population of Los Angeles.

Another way to think about this number is that if we were to try to pack ten billion people into a football field, it would take 263,000 football fields—an area about the size of Houston—to hold them all. Or if ten billion people stood in a line, the line would be two million miles long. That's long enough to reach to the moon and back, four times. It's also long enough to wrap around the entire circumference of the earth eighty times. And we're only talking about the number of animals killed in a single year; consider how these numbers increase over five, ten, twenty years.

Obviously, it takes a lot of animals to produce the amount of meat we, as a nation, buy, sell, and consume. Meat is big business. In fact, meat is very big business—the U.S. animal agribusiness industry has combined annual revenues approaching $125 billion.[8] Consider the countless grocery stores, restaurants, cafeterias, and homes across the country that are stocked with meats. Meat is literally everywhere we turn.

So where are all the animals?

Where Are They?

Of the ten billion animals that have been raised, transported, and slaughtered over the course of the past year, how many have you seen? If you live in a city, probably almost none. But let's assume you live in the country. How many cows do you see grazing on the hillsides? Perhaps fifty at a time, if that? And how about chickens or pigs or turkeys? Do you see any at all? How many times have you seen these animals on television, in magazines and newspapers, in the movies? Though we may eat meat on a daily basis, most of us don't stop to consider how peculiar it is that we can go through our entire lives without ever encountering the animals that become our food. *Where are they?*

The vast majority of the animals we eat are not, as those in the animal agribusiness industry would have us believe, "contented cows" and "happy hens" lazing amid grassy fields and open barnyards. They are not sleeping in spacious stalls with fresh hay. From the moment they are born, these animals are kept in intensive confinement where they may suffer from disease, exposure to extreme temperatures, severe overcrowding, violent handling, and even psychosis. Despite what the prevailing imagery of farm animals suggests, small, family-run farms are largely a thing of the past; today the animals are in massive "confined animal feeding operations," or CAFOs (sometimes called "factory farms"), where they reside until they are shipped to the slaughterhouse.

As with any major production facility, CAFOs (and the slaughterhouses they supply) are designed with a singular intention: to manufacture their product at the lowest cost and for the highest profit possible. Quite simply, the more animals killed per minute, the more money to be made. Toward this end, CAFOs may house literally hundreds of thousands of animals at a time, animals who are viewed and treated as units of production and whose welfare is necessarily secondary to the profit their bodies will turn. From a business standpoint, animal welfare is a *barrier* to profit, as it costs less to mass-produce animals and discard those who die prematurely than it does to care for them adequately. In fact, it is estimated that upwards of 500 million animals destined to become food die before reaching the slaughterhouse, a factor that is built into the cost of production. It is these cost-cutting measures that make modern meat production one of the most inhumane practices in human history.

See No Evil, Hear No Evil, Speak No Evil

The most effective way to distort reality is to deny it; if we tell ourselves there isn't a problem, then we never have to worry about what
to do about it. And the most effective way to deny a reality is to make
it invisible. As we've discussed, invisibility is the bulwark of the carnistic system.

In chapter 2 we deconstructed the *symbolic* invisibility of the
system. Symbolic invisibility is enabled by the defense mechanism
avoidance, which is a form of denial. We avoid the truth when we
avoid naming the system, which, in turn, prevents us from realizing
that there even *is* a system. In this chapter, we will deconstruct the
practical invisibility of carnism. This deconstruction is necessary in
order to truly appreciate the mechanisms and dynamics of carnism.
As long as we are uninformed or misinformed, we cannot understand the reality of meat production and move beyond carnistic
defenses.

The establishments that produce the bulk of the meat that
makes it to our dinner plates are, essentially, invisible. We don't
see them. We don't see them because they are located in remote
areas where most of us don't venture. We don't see them because
we're not allowed access even if we do try to get in.[9] We don't
see them because their trucks are often sealed and unmarked.
We don't see them because, as Erik Schlosser, investigative author of the best-selling *Fast Food Nation,* says, they have "no windows on the front and no architectural clues to what's happening
inside."[10] *We don't see them because we're not supposed to.* As with
any violent ideology, the populace must be shielded from direct
exposure to the victims of the system, lest they begin questioning
the system or their participation in it. This truth speaks for itself:
why else would the meat industry go to such lengths to keep its
practices invisible?

Access Denied

In 2007, journalist Daniel Zwerdling set out to write an article on the chicken industry for *Gourmet* magazine. Given the industry's response to his request for a tour of their plants, one would think Zwerdling was writing for *Vegetarian Times* rather than a renowned publication of carnistic cuisine. According to Zwerdling, whose article "A View to a Kill" was published in the June 2007 issue of *Gourmet,* "Spokesmen at the five biggest companies refused to show me the farms where their suppliers raise the chickens you eat, so that I could see firsthand how they treat them. They refused to show me the slaughterhouses, so I could see how the companies dispatch them. Executives even refused to talk to me about how they raise and kill chickens." And Zwerdling's experience is not uncommon.

Not only is it difficult to obtain access to meatpacking plants, but in a number of states it's actually against the law to take photos or videos inside "animal enterprises," such as laboratories, circuses, and slaughterhouses. Furthermore, the Animal Enterprise Terrorism Act of 2006—legislation that has been harshly criticized as unconstitutional—makes it *illegal to engage in behavior that results in the economic disruption of an animal enterprise.*

Because the media is denied access to "animal enterprises," most of the footage of CAFOs and slaughterhouses that reaches the public comes from undercover investigations. Such was the case with the 2008 Humane Society of the United States (HSUS) investigation that documented workers dragging sick dairy cows with chains and flipping them with forklifts—to be processed into meat destined for public school cafeterias—that led to the largest recall of beef in the nation's history.

This Little Piggy Went to Market . . .

As we discussed in chapter 2, pigs are intelligent, sensitive animals; piglets as young as three weeks old learn their names and respond when called. In fact, research from Pennsylvania State University revealed that pigs could be trained to play computer games; using their snouts to control joysticks, they were able to hit their targets with 80 percent accuracy.[11] Pigs are also affectionate and sociable, enjoying the company of humans, which is why they can make excellent pets. Several years ago, I visited a shelter for rescued farm animals, and the pigs couldn't get enough of my scratching their bellies and behind their ears.

In natural settings, pigs roam for up to thirty miles a day and can form close bonds with one another. They may be able to distinguish between as many as thirty different individual pigs in their group, and will greet and communicate with those with whom they are close. Expectant mothers are extremely conscientious; they may wander for six miles to find the perfect spot to build a birthing nest, and then spend up to ten hours building it before settling in to care for their newborns. Once the babies are old enough to rejoin the others, they play and explore their environment together for months.

Most pigs, however—more than 100 million—spend their entire lives in intensive confinement and never see the outdoors until they are packed into trucks to be sent to slaughter. Shortly after piglets are born, they are typically castrated, and their tails are cut off, without anesthesia. Ranchers are told to remove ("dock") their tails with blunt, side-cutting pliers because the crushing action helps to reduce bleeding. Tail docking is necessary because under extreme stress and when all their natural urges have been thwarted, pigs develop neurotic behaviors and can actually bite each others' tails off. This psychological reaction is one of the symptoms of what is referred to in the industry as porcine stress syndrome (PSS), a condition that is remarkably similar to what we call in humans post-traumatic stress disorder (PTSD). Other symptoms include rigidity, panting, anxiety, blotchy skin, and sometimes sudden death.[12] Like humans who have endured solitary confinement and other tortures in captivity, pigs have engaged in self-mutilation, and have been found repeating the same nonsensical behaviors over and over, sometimes thousands of times a day; the animals are literally driven insane.*

Of Pigs and People: The Genetics of Trauma

Post-traumatic stress disorder (PTSD) and porcine stress syndrome (PSS) seem to share a genetic basis; both conditions are in part hereditary. A number of studies have revealed that one's genetic predisposition, combined with a traumatic experience, increases the likelihood of developing PTSD; a large study of twin Vietnam veterans, for instance, led researchers to claim that there is "a significant genetic contribution to PTSD." Similarly, the Ontario Ministry of Agriculture, Food and Rural Affairs reports that it is the combination of genetics and stress that leads to the development of PSS in pigs.[13]

Piglets born in confinement are allowed to suckle for just two to three weeks, and they do this through the bars of a crate that is separate from their mother's. A number of piglets die before being weaned, from maladies such as starvation or diarrhea. Sometimes if a piglet has managed to squeeze into the mother's crate to satisfy his or her instinctive need for warmth and closeness, the mother

---

*The technical term for repetitive behaviors is *stereotypies*. Stereotypies are a symptom of stress seen in a number of animal species (e.g., large cats pacing in a cage at the zoo), but they are not classified as a symptom of PSS.

can accidentally crush it. Regardless of the cause, infant deaths are inevitable. There are simply too many animals for workers to care for adequately; a typical hog breeding plant employs fifteen people to manage 3,600 sows.

After weaning, for the next six months, the young pigs are crammed into what are often filthy pens or sheds in hog factories. These buildings are filled with noxious gases from the pigs' excrement, and the air is dense with dust and dander. Both pigs and the humans who work in swine confinement buildings suffer from chronic respiratory illnesses, and a number of pigs die prematurely from lung disease.

When the pigs are ready to be slaughtered, they are herded onto tractors bound for the slaughterhouse. To save money, as many pigs as possible are packed into a truck, and this overcrowding—coupled with the fact that the animals receive no food, water, or protection from extreme temperatures during transport, which can last upwards of twenty-eight hours—results in high mortality rates; according to *The National Hog Farmer,* an industry publication, "The national recorded incidence for dead on arrival (DOA) pigs [in 2007] was 0.21%. . . . Based on 22 commercial field trials, the rate of non-ambulatory pigs (classified as fatigued or injured) prior to reaching the weigh scale at the packing plant was about 0.37%. No national figures exist for non-ambulatory pigs."[14] Agricultural investigator Gail Eisnitz, who interviewed a number of slaughterhouse workers, was told of the transport process:

> You're going to lose hogs in a semitrailer no matter what. . . .
> During the time I worked in rendering, there was large piles
> of dead hogs every day. . . . When they come off the truck,
> they're solid as a block of ice. . . . I went to pick up some
> hogs one day for chainsawing from a pile of about thirty fro-
> zen hogs, and I found two [that were] . . . frozen but still
> alive. . . . I could tell they were alive because they raised

their heads up like, "Help me." . . . I took my ax-chopper and chopped them to death.[15]

The pigs that do survive the journey are deposited into holding pens to await slaughter. When it is time, they are prodded onto a narrow walkway, or chute, on which they walk single file to the killing floor. The animals at the rear of the chute hear the screams of the pigs ahead, who have arrived at the slaughter line, as well as the shouts of men working on the noisy production line. Schlosser explains what he saw upon reaching this point in his tour: "The sounds get louder—factory sounds, the noise of power tools and machinery, bursts of compressed air. . . . We walk up a slippery metal stairway and reach a small platform, where the production line begins. A man turns and smiles at me. He wears safety goggles and a hard hat. His face is splattered with gray matter and blood."[16] Not surprisingly, many pigs are reluctant to move forward. As one slaughterhouse worker put it:

> When the hogs smell blood, they don't want to go. I've seen hogs beaten, whipped, kicked in the head to get them up to the restrainer. One night I saw a driver get so angry at a hog he broke its back with a piece of a board. I've seen hog drivers take their prod and shove it up the hog's ass to get them to move. I didn't appreciate that because it made the hogs twice as wild by the time they got to me.[17]

Farm animals are supposed to be stunned and rendered unconscious before they are actually killed. However, some pigs remain conscious when they are strung upside down by their legs in shackles, and they kick and struggle as they are moved along the conveyor belt to have their throats slit. Because of the speed at which the animals are supposed to be stunned and killed, and because slaughterhouse workers are often ineffectively trained, a number of pigs may also survive throat cutting and remain conscious when they arrive at the next station, where they are dropped into scalding water—a procedure done to remove their hair. Eisnitz describes how squealing hogs were left dangling by one leg while workers left to take their lunch breaks, and thousands of hogs were immersed in the scalding tank alive. And one worker she interviewed commented: "These hogs . . . hit the water and start screaming and kicking. Sometimes they thrash so much they kick water out of the tank. . . . There's a rotating arm that pushes them under, no chance for them to get out. I'm not sure if they burn to death before they drown, but it takes them a couple of minutes to stop thrashing."[18]

Eisnitz also found that the stress workers face from spending hours at a single station where they have to kill (or stun) one hog every four seconds led to violent outbursts toward the pigs. One worker described such an incident:

> Like, one day the live hogs were driving me nuts . . . [when] an animal pisses you off [even though you] are going to kill it. . . . Only you don't just kill it, you go in hard, push hard, blow the windpipe, make it drown in its own blood. Split its nose. A live hog would be running around the pit. It would just be looking up at me and I'd be sticking and I would just take my knife and . . . cut its eye out while it was just sitting there. And this hog would just scream. One time I took my knife—it's sharp enough—and I sliced off the end of a hog's nose, just like a piece of bologna. The hog went crazy for a few seconds. Then it just sat there looking kind of stupid. So I took a handful of salt brine and ground it into its nose. Now that hog really went nuts, brushing its nose all over the place. I still had a bunch of salt left on my hand—I was wearing a rubber glove—and I stuck the salt

right up the hog's ass. The poor hog didn't know whether to shit or go blind.[19]

Female pigs that are used as breeders eventually wind up at the slaughterhouse as well, but before that time they spend much of their lives in small metal cages and stalls that are referred to as gestation crates.* These crates are two feet wide, too small for the sows to even turn around, and their floors are covered in feces and urine. The animals suffer from a number of problems due to this confinement, but one of the most painful conditions they endure is urinary tract infections, which can become so severe as to be fatal. Urinary tract infections occur because when the sows lie down, they are immersed in bacteria-ridden waste that makes its way into their urinary tracts. A sow will be forcibly impregnated in rapid cycles of every five or six months, until she is no longer able to reproduce, at which time she is packed onto a truck headed for slaughter.

"Whoever Defines the Issue Controls the Debate"

Timothy Cummings, a poultry veterinarian and clinical professor at Mississippi State University, explained to an audience of poultry producers that it's time to take on media-savvy animal rights activists who understand the power of

---

*Gestation crates have been considered so inhumane that they've been banned in a number of states and nations. The European Union has agreed to phase them out by 2013, and both Smithfield Foods and Maple Leaf Foods, the largest pork producers in the United States and Canada, respectively, said in 2007 that the companies will begin phasing them out as well. Pressure from customers such as McDonald's and Burger King led to the companies' decision.

language. "Whoever defines the issue controls the debate," he said.[20] Cummings suggested that "debeaking" a chicken should instead be called "beak conditioning," making the process seem more like a spa treatment than a disfiguration. The "backup killer" (the worker responsible for slaughtering birds that are still alive after passing the automatic killer) should be a "knife operator," and the term "insanguinated" should replace "bled" to death.

Industry insiders have long been aware of the discomfort consumers feel when words paint too accurate a picture of how animals are turned into meat. As far back as 1922, the Texas Sheep and Goat Raisers' Association proposed replacing "goat meat" with "chevron," arguing that: "People don't eat ground cow, pig chops, or leg of sheep . . . beef, pork, and mutton sound much more appetizing."[21] And the former National Cattlemen's Beef Association advised its members to substitute "process" or "harvest" for "slaughter," since "people react negatively to the word 'slaughtering.'"[22]

In the United Kingdom, too, one can find interesting examples of how the animal agribusiness industry uses language to camouflage the reality of meat. The *Meat Trades Journal* advises readers to use "meat plant" or "meat factory" in lieu of "slaughterhouse."[23] And *British Meat* issued the following statement: "Traditional retailing centres around offering the public bits of animals and often identifies meat with livestock. But modern consumer attitudes shy away from this link. . . . There is an urgent need for a new retailing philosophy. We are no longer in the business of selling pieces of carcase meat. We must make our customers think forward to what they will eat rather than backwards to the animal in the field."[24]

Where's the Beef?

Michael Pollan traced the life of a single steer, steer number 534, in order to write *The Omnivore's Dilemma,* his best-selling exposé on contemporary food-production practices. What Pollan found when he followed steer number 534 from birth to death represents the fate of the 35 million beef cattle that are killed every year in the United States. Pollan describes how he was surveying a herd of calves in a pen when "534 moseyed up to the railing and made eye contact. He had a wide stout frame and was brockle-faced. . . . Here was my boy."[25]

It isn't surprising that 534 so readily approached Pollan. Bovines are communicative, emotional, and social creatures. They have multiple vocalizations and gestures to communicate their feelings, and in a natural environment they will nurture ongoing friendships with one another. Bovines are naturally gentle and docile, spending most of their waking time eating grass and chewing cud. And babies frequently engage in a variety of forms of play with each other when they are not suckling from their mothers.

Bovines born into captivity are unable to satisfy many of these natural instincts. However, for a short time, at least some of their basic needs are met. Unlike the pork and poultry industries, the beef industry keeps its animals outdoors for the first six months of their lives, since it is cheaper to contract independent ranchers who own grazing land to manage this part of the process. Pollan reports: "Steer number 534 spent his first six months in these lush pastures alongside his mother, 9534. . . . Apart from the trauma of the Saturday in April when he was branded and castrated, one could imagine 534 looking back on those six months as the good old days."[26]

Steer 534 had been born in the birthing shed across the street from the pasture, and like all male calves, his castration, branding, and "de-horning" (to prevent his horns from getting stuck in fences or causing harm to other animals or humans) took place without anesthesia. Agriculturalists at the University of Tennessee explain the most efficient ways to perform some of the different methods of castrating calves.[27] Stress from the procedures, they say, can be "minimized by performing the procedure when the calf is small and sexually immature." One method involves using a knife to cut off the lower part of the scrotum: "After the testicles are exposed, they should be grasped and extended one at a time while pushing back the connective tissue surrounding the cord. . . . In young calves, the testicle may be grasped and pulled until the cord breaks." Or operators can place a rubber band on the scrotum above the testicles: "This cuts off the blood supply and the scrotum and testicles slough off in about three weeks." However, they warn, "This is the least desirable of all the bloodless methods of castration because of the danger of tetanus. If this method is used, it should be used on calves less than one month of age." Another bloodless method of castration involves the use of an *emasculatome,* an instrument with blunt blades that crush the spermatic cord and sever the blood supply: "The emasculatome is left in place for approximately one minute. It is strongly suggested that the emasculatome be applied twice on each cord. Repeat the procedure on the other side of the scrotum. . . . If the cord has been missed, repeat the procedure." And finally, the agriculturalists advise that "[t]he best times to castrate are in the spring and fall when flies and maggots are less likely to increase irritation and infection of the wound."

Given these castration practices, it is not surprising that Pollan believes 534 was traumatized. Pollan claims that 534 was traumatized a second time, as well, when he was weaned from his mother at six months of age: "Weaning is perhaps the most traumatic time on a ranch for animals and ranchers alike; cows separated from their calves will bellow for days, and the calves, stressed . . . are prone to getting sick."[28] Weaning is recognized as a major psychological stressor by agricultural veterinarians, who therefore recommend that the facilities that hold both mother and calf after they have been separated should be strong enough to prevent the two from reuniting. The natural suckling period for calves is between six and twelve months.

After weaning, 534 was sent off to spend the next couple of months in a "backgrounding" pen, where he was to get used to confinement, eating from a trough, and consuming unnatural foods, which were comprised of massive quantities of drug-ridden corn, and protein and fat supplements to bring him from 80 to 1,000 pounds in fourteen months. The rest of his life would be spent in a feedlot, an overcrowded, filthy factory farm with flooring largely comprised of manure, where he would be confined with thousands of other steer awaiting slaughter.

When it comes time for slaughter, cattle are no more eager to walk the chute to the kill floor than are pigs. They must be prodded along, a process that further stresses already frustrated animals and workers. Though under federal law it is illegal to use prods in excess of fifty volts, one employee Eisnitz interviewed commented:

> You can get frustrated when you're trying to move cattle along. . . . Sometimes you have to prod them a lot. But some of the drivers [people who prod cattle along the chute] burn the hell out of them. The five or six hotshots (electric prods) by the lead-up chutes are hooked directly to a 110-volt outlet. Run them along the floor's metal grates and they spit sparks like a welding machine. Some drivers would beat cattle with hotshots until they were so wild and panicky you couldn't do a thing with them, right up into the knocking box. . . .[29]

Once at the assembly line, the cattle are stunned, shackled, bled, disemboweled, and skinned. As with hogs, the lack of skilled workers and the dizzying speed of the conveyor belt prevent precision in stunning, and many cattle end up being pulled along while conscious. Conscious cattle on the line are particularly dangerous for workers, because, at 1,000 pounds, when they thrash and kick, they can sometimes break free from the shackles and fall headfirst onto employees from a height of fifteen feet. Even when the animal is directly stunned, sometimes it takes multiple times for the hit to render him unconscious. Another employee comments:

> I remember one bull with really long horns. I knocked it twice. . . . Some solid white stuff came out—brains, I guess—and it went down, its face all bloody. I rolled it into the shackling area. That bull must have felt the shackle going on its leg, it got up like nothing ever happened to it, it didn't even wobble, and took off out the back door, started running down Route 17 and just wouldn't stop. They went out and shot it with a rifle, dragged it back with the tractor.[30]

Schlosser, too, witnessed the effects of inadequate stunning: "A steer slips from its chain, falls to the ground, and gets its head caught in a conveyor belt. The line stops as workers struggle to free the steer, stunned but alive, from the machinery. I've seen enough."[31]

Pollan was not permitted entry to the kill floor, so he awaited the arrival of his steer at the final destination of his journey. There, 534 emerged as a box of steaks. No longer even a number, 534 had been reduced to a container of neatly packaged products destined for supermarket shelves.

They Die Piece by Piece

In 2001, the *Washington Post* printed an article by Joby Warrick entitled "They Die Piece by Piece." Warrick explained how, though cattle were supposed to be dead before reaching the cutting room, this was often not the reality. Ramon

Moreno, a slaughterhouse worker who'd spent twenty years as a "second-legger"—cutting hocks off carcasses as they sped past at the rate of 309 per hour—described the process to Warrick: "'They blink. They make noises,' he said softly. 'The head moves, the eyes are wide and looking around.' Still Moreno would cut. On bad days, he says, dozens of animals reached his station clearly alive and conscious. Some would survive as far as the tail cutter, the belly ripper, the hide puller. 'They die,' said Moreno, 'piece by piece.'"[32]

Bird Brains? Chickens and Turkeys

In chapter 2, I discussed some of the common assumptions we make about pigs and how these beliefs make it easier for us to eat them. Many of us feel even more removed from chickens and turkeys, at least in part because of our deep-rooted belief that they are stupid—perhaps too stupid to even know whether they are in pain. However, birds are actually quite smart; scientists now acknowledge that these animals are vastly more intelligent than they'd realized.[33] Chickens and turkeys are also quite sociable, which may explain the growing trend of keeping them as pets. Owners describe birds who play with them, seek them out for affection, and even cavort with the family dog. There are also websites dedicated exclusively to bird ownership. For instance, at *mypetchicken.com,* enthusiasts can purchase such paraphernalia as the $495 Eglu, an "urban-chic chicken coop," which comes in five different colors, and proud owners can post pictures of their favorite chickens for all to admire.

Nevertheless, in the United States we kill and consume approximately nine billion birds a year for their flesh or eggs. "Broiler" chickens and turkeys are raised for their meat, and though in natural conditions they live up to ten years, in CAFOs they have a life span of seven weeks or sixteen weeks, respectively—which means that, whenever we consume poultry, we are, in fact, eating baby birds. The birds' severely shortened life span is due to their being fed a diet so full of growth-promoting drugs that they grow at a rate that's the equivalent of a human reaching 349 pounds by the age of two. For this reason, meat birds suffer from numerous structural deformities. Their legs are unable to hold their weight and are often twisted and broken; they cannot move much due to chronic joint pain. And when it comes time to be shipped to slaughter, as they are grabbed and crammed into crates that are stacked on top of one another, they can suffer broken or dislocated wings, hips, and legs, as well as internal hemorrhages.

Meat birds spend their lives in barren sheds—or "broiler houses"—that may hold 50,000 birds and be so crowded it is difficult to see the floor. In these conditions, they are unable to carry out any of their natural behaviors, such as foraging and roosting, and the birds develop psychotic, stress-induced behaviors, such as feather pecking and cannibalism. Often, in order to prevent the birds from pecking each other to death, a hot blade is used to cut off the front part of their beaks, without anesthesia, at birth. This procedure, known as debeaking, can lead to infection, the growth of neurological tumors, or death if the bird doesn't have enough of a beak left to use for drinking or eating.

The birds that survive the broiler house are then sent to slaughter. In poultry slaughterhouses, where production speeds are even faster than those for other animals (the average is 8,400 animals per hour), birds are thrown onto conveyors where they are grabbed, sometimes handfuls of them at a time, and hooked upside down on shackles. While the Humane Methods of Slaughter Act requires other animals to be rendered unconscious before being killed, birds are exempt and are slaughtered while fully conscious. Their throats are slit by either hand or machine, and they are then dumped into scalding water to loosen their feathers. A number of birds end up being boiled alive.

Josh Balk, an activist who had worked undercover at a Perdue chicken slaughter plant in 2004 before becoming a director at the Humane Society of the United States, spoke with me about his experience at the plant. He also videotaped and published his accounts of the experience, in particular the workers' ongoing aggression toward the birds. Balk kept a daily log,[34] and following are excerpts:

Nearly every chicken responded with screams and violent physical reactions from the moment they were grabbed by workers and as they went through the line. The screaming of the birds and the frenzied flapping of their wings were so loud that you had to yell to the worker next to you, who was standing less than two feet away, just so he could hear you.

I saw an employee kick a chicken off the floor fan and routinely saw chickens being thrown around the room. . . . While one of the workers was talking about football, he "spiked" a chicken onto the conveyer belt, pretending he had scored a touchdown.

I saw about 50 birds being dumped from the transport crates onto the conveyer belt, a distance of approximately eight feet. The crate tipped them all at once, so they fell on top of each other. The screaming was intense during the whole process. I looked onto the conveyer belt and could clearly see chickens with broken legs and wings, limbs sticking out in unnatural angles.

I . . . noticed that our line leader seemed generally more hostile toward the birds today, even yelling profanities at them when he threw them. . . . During one break, a worker repeatedly slapped a chicken in the face until the line started again.

There were so many dead birds on the floor of the hanging room that it was difficult to take a step without stepping on one.

As with other species destined for human consumption, the American public is shielded from witnessing the lives and deaths of some nine billion chickens per year. As Balk explained, "Being there firsthand to hear the screams and to smell the stench of death in the air is something that most people would never . . . experience."

Can They Suffer?

Calling for the humane treatment of animals, seventeenth-century philosopher Jeremy Bentham argued, "The question is not, 'Can they reason?' nor, 'Can they talk?' but rather, 'Can they suffer?'" The question of sentience—the ability to feel pleasure and pain—has been at the center of arguments surrounding both human and animal welfare.

Historically, members of vulnerable groups have been believed to have a higher tolerance for pain, an assumption often invoked to justify suffering. For instance, fifteenth-century scientists would nail dogs to boards by their paws in order to cut them open and experiment on them while fully conscious, and they dismissed the dogs' howling as simply a mechanical response—as little different from the noise of a clock whose springs have been struck. Similarly, until the early 1980s, American doctors performed major surgery on infants without using painkillers or any anesthetic; the babies' cries were explained as mere instinctive reactions. And because African slaves were thought to feel less pain than whites, it was easier to justify the brutal experience of slavery.

Because the experience of pain is subjective, it is easy to argue against the suffering of another. In other words, since we aren't inside another's body, we can only assume what he or she may be feeling—and if we have a vested interested in assuming that he or she is not in pain, it is all too easy to believe this to be true. Our assumptions stem from our beliefs, and the very belief systems that enable us to inflict suffering on others actively work to keep themselves alive. So it is no wonder that we don't err on the side of caution—or reason—when it comes to carnistic practices that cause animals pain. Consider, for instance, the common assumption that it is nothing more than instinct that drives lobsters to scramble to escape the pot in which they are being boiled alive. Though we have no reason to believe that they are *not* in pain, though it is only logical to assume they are fleeing scalding water because it hurts, and though instinct and sentience can and do coexist (one does not preclude the other), most people choose to believe otherwise.

Objective research is one way to counter our subjective perception of others' experience. Researchers have, for instance, demonstrated that neural pathways in neonates are developed enough for infants to feel pain, and neonates are no longer denied anesthetics. Scientists have also presented sufficient evidence that crustaceans are indeed sentient; some municipalities have therefore made it illegal to boil lobsters alive, and Whole Foods Market, the world's leading organic and natural-food retailer, no longer sells live lobsters or soft-shell crabs on the grounds that their handling and sale is inhumane.

And despite the poultry industry's claims that humans cannot truly know how chickens feel, there is now evidence that strongly suggests birds not only suffer, but actively seek to anesthetize their pain. Researchers took a group of 120 broiler chickens, half of whom were lame, and offered them two types of feed: normal feed and feed that contained an anti-inflammatory painkiller. The lame chickens consumed up to 50 percent more drugged feed than did the nonlame birds and walked better as a result. A second, similar study found that the more severe a chicken's lameness, the more of the drugged feed he consumed. Researchers concluded that the birds were likely self-medicating and that they can, and do, suffer. [35]

Egged On and On: Layer Hens

It is ironic that so many of our "cute" animal pictures—on cards, in calendars, on posters—contain photos of newly born chicks, when every year millions of these baby birds are treated in ways that most of us wouldn't imagine. Layer hens are birds used for egg production. They are born in commercial hatcheries, in industrial incubators. The male chicks are of no economic value and are therefore discarded shortly after birth. They can be dumped into a massive grinder and ground up alive, gassed, or thrown in garbage bins where they die from suffocation or dehydration. The female chicks are stuffed into battery cages, which are wire cages that hold an average of six birds and are about the size of a square filing cabinet.

Hens spend their entire lives in battery cages, where they must eat, sleep, and defecate, and where they cannot even open their wings. The bottoms of the cages are made of wire so that the birds' droppings can fall through the openings, and their limbs can easily become entangled in the mesh. The wires on the sides and top of the cage scrape off the birds' feathers and cause bruises, and some hens neurotically rub their chests against the cage until they are bald and bleeding. Battery cages are considered so cruel that they have already been banned in a number of countries and are being phased out in all twenty-seven nations of the European Union, though they remain widely used throughout the United States.

Because the hens have been genetically manipulated to lay ten times as many eggs as their ancestors, their brittle bones frequently break, as the calcium in their skeletons is disproportionately diverted to eggshell formation. Another consequence of this artificial selection to lay unnaturally large numbers of eggs is uterine prolapse. When an egg gets stuck against the uterine wall, it can pull the uterus out with it. Unless the uterus is pushed back into the hen's body, other hens will peck at it until she bleeds to death or dies of infection; in each case, it usually takes two days for the hen to die.

When they can no longer produce eggs profitably, the hens are pulled out of their cages, sometimes several in a handful, and their limbs, which are weakened and ensnared in the wires, often tear. When she is just over one year old, the layer hen is sent to slaughter.

Death by Wood Chipper: Humane, or Insane?

In 2003, the *LA Times* reported that workers at an egg ranch in San Diego fed "squirming birds by the bucket into [a wood chipper], then turn[ed] the mashed remains with dirt and heap[ed] the mixture into piles." According to the *Times,* veterinarian Gregg Cutler, a member of the animal welfare committee of the American Veterinary Medical Association, authorized the procedure.[36] Prior to the incident, Cutler had been in attendance at a meeting of poultry ranchers discussing how to deal with chickens during an outbreak of Newcastle disease, an avian viral infection. Cutler told the

Times that "[n]o idea was too crazy. We were in desperation trying to deal with this disease." But the 30,000 hens that were being tossed into the wood chipper in San Diego were not infected with Newcastle disease; they had simply stopped producing eggs. Still, according to one of the ranch owners, Cutler and other veterinarians approved the procedure and called it humane. Charges were not pressed against Cutler, and though the San Diego district attorney's office investigated the ranch to assess for animal cruelty, they concluded that there was no evidence of criminal intent on the part of the owners, who were "just following professional advice."

Got Milk? Dairy Cows

Because it is possible to procure milk without harming the cow, most people assume that dairy products are naturally cruelty free. "Naturally" is the operative word here since, like all mass-produced animal foods, contemporary milk production is anything but natural.

Many cows in the United States spend their lives in dairy factories, where they are either chained by the neck and confined within tiny stalls in sheds, or live outdoors in overcrowded, fenced-in feedlots. In the feedlots, the cows eat out of a conveyor belt along a fence, and the ground they stand and lie on is concrete, saturated with urine and feces.

Dairy cows are injected with genetically engineered growth hormones and are artificially impregnated every year, in order to maximize milk production. In most dairies in the United States, the cows are milked by machines for ten months of the year, which includes the seven-month period during which they are pregnant. This process of continual impregnation and lactation stresses their bodies so much that many cows develop lameness and mastitis, an infection and sometimes massive inflammation of the udder. The cow's system is so overworked that her normal metabolic process may be insufficient to keep up with her physical output, and so her natural, herbivorous diet of grazing pasture is supplemented with grain and high-protein, carnivorous feedstuffs made of meat and bonemeal.

Though the physical stress dairy cows endure is significant, it is quite possible that their greatest suffering comes from the emotional trauma they endure each year after giving birth. Their male offspring are used to produce veal, and the females are used for dairy production. As I mentioned earlier, cows are intimately bonded with their calves, whom they may nurse for up to a year. In dairy factories, however, the calf is removed usually within hours of birth so the cow's milk can be diverted for human consumption. Often the calf is dragged away from his or her mother, as the cow bellows hysterically. Other times, to prevent the cow from being provoked, she is taken to another part of the facility to be milked, and the calf is removed in her absence. Like human mothers, cows can become frenzied and desperate when they cannot find their offspring. They will bellow for days, frantically searching for their calves, and sometimes even turning violent, thrashing and kicking at workers. There are even instances of cows escaping and traveling for miles to find their calves on other farms.

Though cows have a natural life span of approximately twenty years, after only four years in a dairy factory they are considered spent and are sent to slaughter. A significant proportion of U.S. ground beef is made from dairy cows.

Out of the Mouths of Babes: Veal

Many people have a soft spot for babies, bovines notwithstanding. Most of us are touched by the sight of a newborn calf entering the world, and sympathize with his or her innocence, fragility, and vulnerability. In fact, wobbly-legged calves are often favorites of children's books. Imagine, then, the shock of many Americans when they learn of the plight of the approximately one million calves a year who are the unwanted by-products of the dairy industry. In fact, if it weren't for the dairy industry, the veal industry would likely not exist.

Because male calves born to dairy cows are of no use to dairy farmers, they are essentially disposed of. Days or even hours after birth, the calves are herded onto a truck, and some need to be dragged since they may not yet be able to walk properly. These calves end up at auctions, where they may be sold for as little as $50 to veal producers. And since they are literally newborns, it is not unusual for calves in the auction ring to have hides still slick from the womb and umbilical cords dangling from their stomachs.

For the duration of their short lives—though some are killed within days, most veal calves live for sixteen to eighteen weeks—they are chained or tethered at the neck and confined to stalls so tiny they can't even turn around or lie down normally.[*][37] And in order to produce the pale color that veal is known for, the animals are typically fed an unnatural diet lacking in iron, so that they are in a state of chronic borderline anemia. Veal calves spend their lives immobilized and sickly, and not surprisingly, they have been observed to exhibit some of the same neurotic behaviors as other animals under intense stress: abnormal head tossing and scraping, kicking, scratching, and chewing.

The slaughter of calves is no different than the slaughter of other animals; they are meant to be stunned before being shackled, but

*Spokespersons for the veal industry say the industry intends to phase out individual calf stalls and transition to group pens by 2017.

again, this method is far from perfect. A worker that Eisnitz interviewed describes a part of the process:

> In the morning the big holdup was the calves. . . . To get done with them faster, we'd put eight or nine of them in the knocking box at a time. As soon as they start going in, you start shooting, the calves are jumping, they're all piling up on top of each other. You don't know which ones got shot and which ones didn't get shot at all, and you forget to do the bottom ones. They're hung anyway, and down the line they go, wriggling and yelling. The baby ones—two, three weeks old—I felt bad killing them so I just let them walk past.[38]

There seems to be a point at which the violence of carnism is such that even the most powerful defenses of the system will falter.

Sea Food, or Sea Life? Fish and Other Sea Animals

Many of us feel so removed from fish and other commonly consumed creatures of the sea that we don't even think of their flesh as meat. For instance, when a carnist learns that someone is vegetarian, the carnist will often respond by asking, "So, you only eat fish?" We tend not to perceive sea creatures' flesh as meat because—though we know they're neither plants nor minerals—we often don't think of sea creatures as animals. And by extension, we don't think of these beings as sentient, as having lives that matter to them. We thus relate to the animals of the sea as if they were anomalous plants, plucking them from the ocean as easily as we pluck an apple from a tree.

But are sea animals the mindless, insensate organisms many of us assume them to be? Not according to a number of neurobiologists, animal behaviorists, and other scientists around the world. There is a significant body of research demonstrating that fish and other creatures of the sea possess both intelligence and the capacity to feel pain. Research on the intelligence of sea life has, for example, yielded evidence that fish do not forget what they've experienced just moments before, but have a memory span of at least three months.[39] Moreover, Oxford University scientist Dr. Theresa Burt de Perera determined that fish can develop "mental maps" of their surroundings that allow them to memorize and navigate changes in their environment—a task that is beyond the cognitive ability of hamsters. Because of such findings, it is now illegal in the city of Monza, Italy, to keep goldfish confined in small bowls. And lobsters, some of which have a life span longer than that of humans, possess over 400 types of chemical receptors on their antennae which, according to Dr. Jelle Atema of the Marine Biological Laboratory in Woods Hole, Massachusetts, may enable them to detect the sex, species, and even mood of another animal.

I pointed out earlier in this chapter that scientists have demonstrated the sentience of some types of crustaceans such that legislation has been passed protecting these species. Similarly, evidence that other sea animals can feel pain is amassing; for instance, researchers have found that fish have a number of pain receptors in various parts of their bodies, and they emit neurotransmitters that act as pain killers much as human endorphins do.[40] In one study, researchers from the Roslin Institute and the University of Edinburgh injected the lips of one group of fish with a painful, acidic substance and they injected the lips of another group with saline. The first group of fish exhibited a rocking motion "strikingly similar to the kind of motion seen in stressed . . . mammals." Moreover, the animals were clearly suffering: they rubbed their lips on the gravel in their tank and against the tank walls, and didn't resume feeding for almost three times longer than the control group. (This study has spurred the debate about the ethics of recreational fishing, with animal advocates arguing that impaling fish in their mouths for fun is a form of animal cruelty.)

Other research has suggested that sea animals may actually experience a post-traumatic reaction to pain. In a landmark study, scientists from Purdue University and the Norwegian School of Veterinary Science attached foil heaters to two groups of fish, and administered morphine to one group. They raised the temperature of the foil to observe the reaction of the fish (no fish were permanently harmed in the experiment). The researchers assumed that the morphine would enable the fish to withstand more heat. As it turned out, both groups of fish wriggled at the same temperature, leading the researchers to conclude that the wriggling was a reflexive reaction and didn't indicate pain. However, after the fish had been returned to their tanks, those that hadn't been given morphine exhibited defensive behaviors, indicating anxiety or wariness. The researchers determined that the fish were having a post-traumatic response to the pain: "They turned that pain into fear like we do."

Nevertheless, in the United States, ten billion sea animals are slaughtered each year, many of which are destined for human consumption. There are two ways that these animals are captured, raised, and killed: by commercial fishing and through aquatic farming.[41] Each of these methods causes intensive suffering to the animals and extensive damage to the environment.

Commercial fishing is responsible not only for the depletion of 70 percent of the world's fish species, but also for serious injury to other species of animals. One method used to catch fish is by dragging long nets beneath the surface of the ocean. These nets result in massive amounts of "bycatch"— captured animals other than those targeted. It is estimated that each year, over 30 million tons of sea animals, including birds, turtles, dolphins, and unwanted fish, are thrown back into the ocean, dead or dying; nets left at sea continue to ensnare seabirds and other animals that unwittingly encounter them. Some fisheries use dynamite or cyanide in lieu of nets, but such methods can destroy entire ecosystems. Commercial fishing poses such a threat to marine biodiversity that it's been referred to as "underwater clear-cutting."

Some people choose to eat farm-raised fish rather than commercially caught fish to help preserve the oceans' biodiversity. However, most of the feed used for farm-raised fish comes from the sea; it is estimated that for every pound of farmed fish produced, up to five pounds of marine life are used. Farmed fish are raised in aquafarms, which are CAFOs for sea animals. These facilities can be either land based, in controlled, indoor environments, or ocean based, situated close to the shoreline. Both types of aquafarms hold tens of thousands of fish or other sea animals packed into overcrowded pens that are rife with parasites and disease. To control for illness, accelerate growth, and modify reproductive behaviors, the animals are given antibiotics, pesticides, and hormones and some are genetically modified. The chemicals are absorbed by the animals and also leech out into the environment, ending up in our digestive systems and our ecosystem. It is not uncommon for fish to escape from ocean-based pens, and when they do, they may spread disease or reproduce and contaminate the gene pool.

Fish may be slaughtered in a number of ways. Commercially caught fish are often left to suffocate to death after being landed. Farmed fish are typically removed from their pens by a pump, and dumped into a slaughter area. There, various slaughter methods may be applied, including electrocution, which leads to a lethal, epileptic-like seizure; percussive stunning, which is administering a blow to the head with a club; live chilling, in which the animals are left on ice and frozen alive; suffocation; or spiking, where a spike is inserted through the animals' brain.

Despite the violence inherent in the production of sea food, many people are undisturbed by the sight of at least some aspects of this process. So the primary defense of the carnistic system, invisibility, plays a lesser role when it comes to processing sea creatures; most people can witness fish slaughter, for instance, without experiencing the trauma they might feel witnessing the slaughter of a pig. It would seem that, because sea animals appear so fundamentally different from humans, so alien, we feel sufficiently distanced from them so that their suffering remains invisible even when it's in plain sight.

On Death's Door: Downed Animals

Downed animals, or "nonambulatory livestock," are (land) animals that are too sick or injured to stand up or walk on their own. They are often left to die of neglect at stockyards and auctions. Still-living animals have been documented being dumped onto a "dead pile," which may contain dozens of corpses. The downed animals that are not discarded may be dragged by hooks or chains or bulldozed by a forklift, a process that severely injures already crippled animals.[42] (In 2004, after the first case of mad cow disease was reported in the United States, the USDA banned the practice of using some, though not all, downed cattle for human consumption. And in March 2009, President Barack Obama announced that the USDA would move toward banning all nonambulatory cattle from being used in the nation's food supply.)

In violent ideologies, not only is the violence itself invisible, so, too, are its remains. Where are all the "leftovers" of meat production? Where are the piles and piles of downed animals, the upwards of 500 million animals that may be thrown atop one another and left to die?

"This Obscene . . . Torture Has Got to Stop, and Only People Like Us Can Help."

In South Korea, millions of dogs are killed for their meat every year. While the Korean dog-meat trade is not officially sanctioned by the government, neither is it reprehended. Currently, legislation is being drafted that would classify dogs as livestock, a move that could cause the dog-meat industry to mushroom.

In 2002, the British *Telegraph* published an article documenting the lives and deaths of the dogs raised for their meat:

> The stench and the yelps of caged dogs may be stomach churning, but Lee Wha-jin happily slaps down dishes of dog-meat stew on the white plastic tabletops of his restaurant in the notorious Moran night market in Seoul.
>
> At the rear of shop after shop, eight-month-old puppies—considered to be the prime age for eating—are packed into tiny cages welded together in rows three or four high.
>
> Customers choose which of the live animals they want. The dog is then taken to the back of the shop where a flimsy curtain or a swinging door obscures the sight, but not the sound, of a hideous death. . . .
>
> Before arriving in the grim array of cages behind restaurants, most dogs have had to endure the misery of a Korean canine farm hidden in the hills of

the countryside. It is not unusual for puppies to grow up 10 to a cage, covered in sores and lice. . . .

The dogs' deaths are as inhumane as their rearing. The majority are beaten to death, as it is thought to stimulate the production of adrenalin that South Korean men believe will bolster their virility.

Once dead, or nearly dead, the dogs are dropped into boiling water, skinned and hung by the jaw from a meat hook. Many cooks then use a blow torch to glaze the carcass.[43]

The South Korean dog-meat trade has been met with violent opposition from animal advocacy groups and foreigners—many of whom regularly consume the meat of pigs, chickens, and bovines. Lee Won-Bok, president of the Korea Association for Animal Protection, says, "It's horrible to imagine dog meat on display next to beef and ham at supermarkets." And horrified bloggers on the American Society for the Prevention of Cruelty to Animals (ASPCA)'s website[44] echo his sentiment. Like Won-Bok, the bloggers give voice to what many people feel when they become aware of animal cruelty:

[D]ecent people can not bring themselves to confront this issue because of the sheer and utter horror food and fur dogs/cats etc. go through in the far east, millions of dogs and cats are skinned alive, boiled alive, some even skinned alive THEN boiled alive. [T]he far east is responsible for the worst, most obscene cruelty towards animals this planet has ever seen, and it's on a vast scale.

. . . [M]ost people only see and hear what they want to and that because this isn't taking place here in the USA that people will tend to ignore it but just because this is happening overseas it won't go away. People need to get their heads out of the sand and stand up for these animals.

For dogs that are eventually killed for consumption, if they even have a life, it is a life of sheer misery. . . . Dogs are neither wild animals nor livestock. . . . Everyone all over the world must act now. Save dogs in Korea. We believe you can.

[I']ve seen cruelty from all around the world, but the far east is truly shocking in its attitude towards animals . . . why is this? [M]y theory is cos *[sic]* they know the enlightened west generally give dogs/cats the respect they deserve, and their backward societys *[sic]* are unwilling to catch up.
    [I] gather that many [people] are utterly ignorant of the situation in the Far East, and to be honest you can not really blame them, after all, how many decent people would even dream that animals could be subjected to such unnecessary alien cruelty.

[D]ecent people everywhere have to confront this issue, despite the fact it will give them nightmares. . . . [T]his obscene satanic devlish *[sic]* torture has got to stop, and only people like us can help.

If Slaughterhouses Had Glass Walls

Sir Paul McCartney once claimed that if slaughterhouses had glass walls, everyone would be vegetarian. He believed that if we knew the truth about meat production, we'd be unable to continue eating animals.

Yet on some level we do know the truth. We know that meat production is a messy business, but we choose not to know just how messy it is. We know that meat comes from an animal, but we choose not to connect the dots. And often, we eat animals and choose not to know we're even making a choice. Violent ideologies are structured so that it is not only possible, but inevitable, that we are aware of an unpleasant truth on one level while being oblivious to it on another. Common to all violent ideologies is this phenomenon of *knowing without knowing*. And it is the essence of carnism.

Inherent in violent ideologies is an implicit contract between producer and consumer to see no evil, hear no evil, and speak no evil. Sure, animal agribusinesses go to great lengths to protect their secrets. But we make their job easy for them. They tell us not to look, and we turn away. They tell us the billions of animals that we never see live outdoors on peaceful farms, and as illogical as this is, we don't question it. We make their job easy because on some level most of us don't want to know the way things really are.

But at the same time, we also want and deserve the freedom to make informed decisions, to be free thinkers and active consumers. Such freedom is obviously impossible if we aren't even aware that we are making choices in the first place. When an invisible ideology guides our beliefs and behaviors, we become casualties of a system that has stolen our freedom to think for ourselves and to act accordingly.

When we understand the way things really are—when we recognize the inner workings of the system—then, and only then, are we in a position to make our choices freely. Naming carnism and de-mystifying the practices of meat production can help us begin to see through the façade of the system. Schlosser eloquently expresses this point, and it seems only fitting to end this chapter with the conclusion of his journey through the lives and deaths of the animals we eat:

> As I walk along the fence, a group of cattle approaches me, looking me straight in the eye, like dogs hoping for a treat, and follow me, out of some mysterious impulse. I stop and try to absorb the whole scene: the cool breeze, the cattle and their gentle lowing, a cloudless sky, steam rising from the [meat] plant in the moonlight. And then I notice that the building does have one window, a small square of light on the second floor. It offers a glimpse of what's hidden behind this huge, blank façade. Through the little window you can see bright-red carcasses on hooks, going round and round.[45]

CHAPTER 4

COLLATERAL DAMAGE:
THE OTHER CASUALTIES
OF CARNISM

Facts do not cease to exist because they are ignored.
—Aldous Huxley

In chapter 3 we explored the lives and deaths of the animals most commonly raised for meat, eggs, and dairy products in the United States. For the sake of brevity, I did not discuss the less frequently consumed animals, such as lambs, goats, and ducks. I also didn't mention an important group of animals that are the other casualties of carnism, animals that are the all-too-often-overlooked *collateral damage* of animal agribusiness.

Like pigs and other species we have discussed, the vast majority of these animals—over 300 million of them—are treated as commodities, as means to ends. Like the other animals, their welfare impedes profit. And like the other animals, they are offered little protection by the law.

These other casualties of carnism are rarely the focus of attention when discussing meat production. They, too, are invisible victims—not because they are not seen, but because they are not recognized. They are the human animals. They are the factory workers, the residents who live near polluting CAFOs, the meat consumers, the taxpayers. They are you and I. *We* are the collateral damage of carnism;

we pay for it with our health, our environment, and our taxes—$7.64 billion a year, to be exact.[46]

Workers in meatpacking plants spend virtually all of their waking hours in crowded factories with floors that may be covered in blood and grease.[47] The relentless pace of the disassembly line keeps them at constant risk of serious injury. And CAFO employees—who are exposed to noxious gases from concentrated wastes—may develop serious respiratory disease, reproductive dysfunction, neurological degeneration, seizures, and comas.[48] Such congested and dangerous working conditions can lead to a variety of other physical maladies, but these employees rarely receive medical treatment since it is more cost effective to lose some of them prematurely than to attend to their physical needs. Not surprisingly, like other animals that must be prodded along when they resist following orders, workers in animal factories may be bullied, both physically and psychologically, if they fail to respond to demands.

Residents who live near CAFOs have been poisoned by factory wastes, including sulfites and nitrates. These toxins contaminate the air and drinking water and can lead to chronic asthma and eye irritation, bronchitis, diarrhea, severe headaches, nausea, spontaneous abortions, birth defects, infant death, and viral and bacterial disease outbreaks.

And meat consumers—roughly 300 million Americans—are unknowingly fed an array of contaminants. Our meat is often laced with synthetic hormones, some of which have been linked to the development of various cancers and are banned from both human and animal consumption in the European Union; massive doses of antibiotics; toxic pesticides, herbicides, and fungicides that are known carcinogens; potentially deadly strains of bacteria and viruses; petroleum; poisoned rat carcasses; dirt; hair; and feces.[49]

In his best-selling *Fast Food Nation*, Eric Schlosser captures the essence of the collateral damage of carnism: "There's shit in the meat."

Yet while Schlosser was referring specifically to fecal matter, the subject of this chapter includes far more than just feces. It's everything that contaminates the meat we eat, from corruption to disease. It is the refuse of a sick system.

The story of how shit got in our meat is the story of one of the central characteristics of carnism, and of other violent ideologies: the system depends on a constituency of *indirect* victims, inadvertent victims who not only suffer the consequences of the system, but who also help that system by unwittingly participating in their own victimization. The system creates such victims by appearing to be something it is not, so that we feel safe when we are at risk and free when we have been coerced. The story of how shit got in our meat is the story of the human casualties of carnism.

How Safe Are We?

In 1906, Upton Sinclair published *The Jungle,* his famous exposé on the meatpacking industry. *The Jungle* documented the corruption of animal agribusinesses and the filthy, dangerous conditions that characterized meatpacking plants and slaughterhouses. Sinclair described factories where workers stood in half an inch of blood, on killing floors teeming with rats—living and dead—some of which ended up processed along with the meat. The workers were at constant risk of getting their fingers sliced off and of falling into vats of lard, "overlooked for days, till all but the bones of them had gone out to the world as Durham's Pure Leaf Lard!"[50] *The Jungle* exposed conditions so appalling and disgusting that citizens and policymakers alike were outraged. Such public indignation led to the passage of the Meat Inspection Act and the Pure Food and Drug Act, which mandated regular inspections of slaughterhouses and meatpacking plants.

Many people have heard of *The Jungle* and its impact on laws regulating meat production. However, few realize that these laws were rarely enforced, and that the decades following the publication of *The Jungle* saw little improvement in factory conditions. In fact, in many ways, today conditions are even worse; the advent of larger plants and faster processing technologies, coupled with inadequate numbers of federal inspectors, have made workers more burdened and facilities even more crowded and difficult to police.

Infections, Inspections, and the USDA

Inspections take place on two levels: up close and from a distance. In accordance with the Meat Inspection Act of 1906, USDA inspectors were to perform up-close inspections: they were to check animals' organs and other body parts for disease, equipment for microbes, carcasses for early signs of contamination and insects, and walls and rooms for proper sanitation. However, in the 1980s, new legislation shifted the burden of quality control from the government to the plants themselves.[51] This means that the corporations' own employees, rather than federal inspectors, are now primarily responsible for the closer inspections—employees who have been found to lack the education and experience to identify many of the signs of contamination and disease, and who often don't speak English well enough to communicate what they do find. Since the passing of the new legislation, studies in several plants revealed that corporate inspectors didn't know that a piece of meat that had a USDA tag on it was condemned, and they couldn't recognize the signs of measles. These investigations also revealed that corporate inspectors were unable to recognize infections unless there was pus oozing out of an abscess. In fact, it appears that in our nation's meatpacking plants, contaminated meat is the rule, rather than the exception; researchers from the University of Minnesota found that in over a thousand food samples from numerous retail markets, 69 percent of the pork and beef and 92 percent of the poultry were contaminated with fecal matter that contained the potentially dangerous bacterium *E. coli*, and according to a recent study published in the *Journal of Food Protection* fecal contamination was found in 85 percent of fish fillets procured from retail markets and the Internet.[52] What's more, the World Health Organization has warned that avian influenza—the potentially deadly virus sometimes referred to as "bird flu"—may be spread through the fecal matter of infected birds.[53]

Even if workers were able to identify contaminated body parts, food-quality standards are so low that many defective carcasses would still pass inspection. Carcasses have been considered acceptable for human consumption even when they've contained blood clots, stains, scar tissue from ulcers, liver spots, and hemorrhages. As one USDA inspector explained, "Veterinarians are now approving cattle that wheeze loudly as they're breathing before slaughter and whose lungs are filled with fluid, that have scar tissue and abscesses running all up and down the sides of the lungs, and stuck to their ribs, and have popped blood vessels in kidneys that are no longer functional . . . that are stuffed with regurgitated food . . . oozing out."[54] And in 2007, the *Chicago Tribune* ran an article exposing how the USDA deemed it acceptable for animal agribusinesses to sell meat that's been contaminated with *E. coli,* as long as the meat was labeled "cook only." Cook-only meat is supposedly safe to eat as long as it's been thoroughly cooked, and—unbeknownst to consumers—it's been sold as precooked meat products and has ended up in school lunches.[55]

Unhygienic conditions of the buildings and machinery may also pose a threat to human health. A 2001–2002 review of USDA reports by Human Rights Watch revealed a failure of Nebraska Beef, one of the nation's largest meatpacking companies, to meet basic sanitation standards. Apart from documenting contamination of carcasses, including "visible ingesta [food from an animal's digestive tract] on . . . carcass sides; visible fecal material on the neck, armpit, underneath the foreshanks, and underneath the brisket area of two carcass sides; an 11″ x 1″ fecal contamination smear above the shoulder (of a carcass); several pieces of a greenish fecal matter in the belly area," the review noted the following conditions: "a closed rat trap contained a decomposed mouse . . . a backed up floor drain with a grayish and black residue buildup on floor . . . black splattering on boxes of edible product . . . smelled of sewage . . . no rodent windup trap checks during pest control inspection; visible yellow ingesta behind the stainless steel shield. . . ."[56]

It is perhaps not surprising, then, that Nebraska Beef eventually ended up recalling its ground beef—nearly 550,000 pounds of it. The recall took place in June 2008, after fifty people had fallen ill from eating meat that was contaminated with *E. coli*. After the recall, federal authorities assured consumers that the company's meat was safe to consume. Yet less than a month later, another outbreak caused Nebraska Beef to recall 1.2 million pounds of contaminated beef.[57]

Some USDA inspectors have expressed grave concern about the unhygienic conditions in meat plants, and yet they have little voice to enact change. They no longer have the authority to stop the line if they notice something suspicious, nor can they take remedial action. In fact, in order for a federal inspector's complaint to be seriously considered, the company *itself* must agree that there is a problem.

The vast inadequacies of the current inspection system were described in another 2007 *Chicago Tribune* article.[58] Felicia Nestor, a senior policy analyst for Food and Water Watch, a Washington, DC–

based food safety group, told the *Tribune:* "Inspectors are not . . . in the vast majority of processing plants full time. . . . For the most part, inspectors at processing plants are on patrols, meaning they cover a number of plants." And federal officers reported that inspection goals haven't been met for years; their workload is so overwhelming that they perform mere cursory checks of company records, rather than conduct physical examinations of meat and eggs. Inspectors spend their time monitoring a meat company's hazard-analysis plan and have no time to actually enforce the USDA's inspection regulations. One inspector told the *Tribune,* "They [meatpacking companies] write their own plan. They write everything for themselves. We're 'monitoring' that now. It's just a joke. We mostly check paper now. You can put anything you want on paper."

What this all comes down to is that corporations, whose primary objective is to increase their profit margin, are left to police themselves. We have left the fox to guard the chicken coop. And not surprisingly, we have ended up with shit in our meat.

The Human Slaughterhouse Animal

Meat has long stood for the freedom to exploit freely.
—Nick Fiddes, **Meat: A Natural Symbol**

Many workers in meatpacking plants are undocumented immigrants from Latin America and Asia who receive little, if any, training. Schlosser interviewed a bleeder (slaughterhouse worker) who told him, "Nobody helped train me—no training how to use the knife. . . . So you see how the people on either side of you do the work, and then you do it."[59] Besides having to perform jobs for which they are wholly unprepared, these employees find themselves in working conditions that are exploitative, hazardous, unsanitary, and violent. They spend hour upon hour in a death-saturated, high-stress environment, and they suffer for it—imagine killing twenty-three chickens per minute, totaling *twenty-five thousand* a day.

In an interview with *Mother Jones* magazine, Schlosser comments on the relentless pace of the production line:

> The golden rule in meatpacking plants is "The Chain Will Not Stop." . . . Nothing stands in the way of production, not mechanical failures, breakdowns, accidents. Forklifts crash, saws overheat, workers drop knives, workers get cut, workers collapse and lie unconscious on the floor, as dripping carcasses sway past them, and the chain keeps going . . . a . . . worker told me, "I've seen bleeders, and they're gushing because they got hit right in the vein, and I mean they're almost passing out, and here comes the supply guy again, with the bleach, to clean the blood off the floor, but the chain never stops. It never stops."[60]

Not surprisingly, meatpacking is the single most dangerous factory job in the United States, and it is also the most violent. For instance, workers must wear hockey masks to prevent their teeth from getting kicked out by conscious animals being dragged along a conveyor belt. And consider the titles of accident reports issued by the federal Occupational Safety and Health Administration (OSHA), which provide snapshots of the perilous conditions: *Employee Hospitalized for Neck Laceration from Flying Blade. Employee's Eye Injured When Struck by Hanging Hook. Employee's Arm Amputated When Caught in Meat Tenderizer. Employee Decapitated by Chain of Hide Puller Machine. Employee Killed When Head Crushed in Hide Fleshing Machine. Caught and Killed by Gut-Cooker Machine.*[61] In fact, in 2005, for the first time ever, Human Rights Watch

issued a report criticizing a single U.S. industry—the meat industry—
for working conditions so appalling they violate basic human rights.[62]

Operational Hazards in the Meatpacking Industry

Operation Performed	Equipment/ Substances	Accidents/ Injuries
Stunning	Knocking gun	Severe shock, body punctures
Skinning/removing front legs	Pincher device	Amputations, eye injuries, cuts, falls
Splitting animal	Splitter saws	Eye injury, carpal tunnel syndrome, amputations, cuts, falls
Removing brain	Head splitter	Cuts, amputations, eye injury, falls
Transporting products	Screw conveyers, screw auger	Fractures, cuts, amputations, falls
Cutting/trimming/ boning	Hand knives, saws— circular saw, band saw	Cuts, eye injuries, carpal tunnel syndrome, falls
Removing jaw bone/ snout	Jaw bone/snout puller	Amputations, falls
Preparing bacon for slicing	Bacon/belly press	Amputations, falls
Tenderizing	Electrical meat tenderizers	Severe shock, amputations, cuts, eye injuries
Cleaning equipment	Lock-out, tag-out	Amputations, cuts
Hoisting/shackling	Chain/dolly assembly	Falls, falling carcasses
Wrapping meat	Sealant machine/polyvinyl chloride, meat	Exposure to toxic substances, severe burns to hands and arms, falls
Lugging meat	Carcasses	Severe back and shoulder injuries, falls
Refrigeration/curing, cleaning, wrapping	Ammonia, carbon dioxide, carbon monoxide, polyvinyl chloride	Upper respiratory irritation and damage

Source: Publication of the U.S. Department of Labor, Occupational and Safety Health Administration (OSHA)

Conditioned Killers

Given the brutality of the slaughter process, it is easy to assume that the people whose job it is to kill animals are sadistic or otherwise psychologically disturbed. Yet while psychological disturbance and even sadism may *result* from prolonged exposure to violence, they do not necessarily *cause* individuals to seek out a career in killing. In any violent ideology, those in the business of killing may not be jaded when they start out, but they eventually grow accustomed to violence that once disturbed them. Such acclimation reflects the defense mechanism *routinization*—routinely performing an action until one becomes desensitized, or numbed, to it. For instance, agricultural investigator Gail Eisnitz interviewed a slaughterhouse worker who told her:

> The worst thing, worse than the physical danger, is the emotional toll. If you work in that stick pit for any period of time, you develop an attitude that lets you kill things but doesn't let you care. You may look a hog in the eye that's walking around down in the blood pit with you and think, "God, that really isn't a bad-looking animal." You may want to pet it. Pigs down on the kill floor have come up and nuzzled me like a puppy. Two minutes later, I had to kill them—beat them to death with a pipe. I can't care.[63]

And the more desensitized workers become—the more they "can't care"—the greater the buildup of their psychological distress. Most people can experience only so much violence before they become traumatized by it; studies of combat veterans, for instance, demonstrate again and again the profound effect exposure to violence has on the psyche, particularly when one has also been a participant in that violence. Traumatized workers become increasingly violent toward both animals and humans, and develop addictive behaviors in an attempt to numb their distress. The worker Eisnitz interviewed described how he'd "had ideas of hanging [the] foreman upside down on the line and sticking him."[64] This worker went on to explain:

> Most stickers have been arrested for assault. A lot of them have problems with alcohol. They have to drink, they have no other way of dealing with killing live, kicking animals all day long. . . . A lot of guys . . . just drink and drug their problems away. Some of them end up abusing their spouses because they can't get rid of the feelings. They leave work with this attitude and they go down to the bar to forget. Only problem is, even if you try to drink those feelings away, they're still there when you sober up.[65]

Another worker told Eisnitz:

> I've taken out my job pressure and frustration on the animals. . . . [T]here was a live hog in the pit. It hadn't done anything wrong, wasn't even running around the pit. It was just alive. I took a three-foot chunk of pipe—and I literally beat that hog to death. Couldn't have been a two-inch piece of solid bone left in its head. Basically, if you want to put it in layman's terms, I crushed his skull. It was like I started hitting the hog and I couldn't stop. And when I finally did stop, I'd expended all this energy and frustration, and I'm thinking, what in God's sweet name did I do?[66]

And an undercover video shot by People for the Ethical Treatment of Animals reveals workers slamming piglets onto the floor, bragging about stabbing rods into sows' hindquarters, and hitting pigs with metal rods. As one worker hits a sow with a metal rod, he yells, "I hate them. These (expletives) deserve to be hurt. Hurt, I say! Hurt! Hurt! Hurt! Hurt! . . . Take out your frustrations on 'em."[67]

Though the behavior of meat packers may seem extreme and irrational, it is the inevitable result of working on the front lines of an extreme and irrational system.* Traumatized workers that, in turn, traumatize others are yet another casualty of the violent ideology that is carnism. Violence does indeed beget violence.

The Untouchables

Most people, whether they eat meat or not, share the same attitude toward the slaughtering of animals: they see the process as disgusting and offensive. Just as a type of meat that one finds disgusting tends to render the foods it touches disgusting as well (would you continue eating a stew you'd picked dog meat out of?), so, too, does the process of slaughter seem to contaminate those who butcher animals.[68]

In various cultures and throughout history, professional butchers have been seen as impure, as taking on the immorality of killing animals and thereby protecting others from moral contamination. Often a group will have a designated individual or individuals who perform the butchering, and they either will be "morally cleansed" before coming into contact with the others, or will live separately from the rest of the community. For instance, the designated butcher of the Bemba of Northern Rhodesia performs purification ceremonies after butchering, and the butchers of the ancient

---

*Some slaughterhouse workers no doubt enter the industry as sociopaths: individuals who are antisocial, clinically "conscienceless," and often take pleasure in causing others to suffer. However, one must wonder at an industry that tolerates—indeed, *requires*—antisocial behaviors such as extreme aggression, remorselessness, and violence.

Guanches of the Canary Islands weren't allowed to enter others' homes or associate with those who weren't also butchers. In some cases, an entire social group is assigned the task of butchering: in Japan, for instance, butchers have been members of the Eta, an underclass whose members have been prevented from having contact with others; in India the Untouchables have been considered spiritually inferior and so have been relegated to spiritually "polluting" tasks such as butchering and working with leather; and in Tibet, professional butchers have been members of the lowest classes, because they violate the Buddhist tenet against killing.

Our Planet, Our Selves

Even if you don't work in the meatpacking industry or eat meat, you are not immune to the consequences of the practices of the animal agribusinesses with which you share the planet. Meat production is a leading cause of every significant form of environmental damage: air and water pollution, biodiversity loss, erosion, deforestation, greenhouse gas emissions, and depletion of fresh water.[69]

In the industrialized world, the most immediate environmental consequence of meat production is the pollution caused by CAFOs. Mounds of chemical- and disease-ridden waste produced by these factories leach into the ground and waterways and evaporate into the air, toxifying the environment and sickening the humans who reside nearby. CAFO runoff has been linked with a number of maladies, including respiratory problems, severe headaches, and digestive disorders. CAFO waste has also been connected with spontaneous abortions, birth defects, infant death, and disease outbreaks. In fact, CAFOs pose such a hazard to human health that the U.S. Department of Public Health has urged a moratorium on their toxic dumping.[70]

Yet animal agribusinesses have continued their practices unremittingly—because they can. Even though they are systematically destroying the environment and the people in it, animal agribusinesses aren't breaking any laws. How is it that the legal system, which was established to protect us from exploitation, ends up instead protecting the very industries that exploit us? Whatever happened to democracy?

The Environmental Costs of Meat[71]

- The United Nations has declared the livestock sector "one of the top two or three most significant contributors to the most serious environmental problems, at every scale from local to global. The impact is so significant" they warn, "that it needs to be addressed with urgency."

- Animal agriculture is likely the world's largest source of water pollution. The main sources of the pollution are from antibiotics and hormones, chemicals from tanneries, animal wastes, sediments from eroded pastures, and fertilizers and pesticides used for feed crops.

- Seventy percent of previously forested land in the Amazon is now pastures for feeding livestock.

- Livestock-based agribusiness causes 55 percent of the erosion and sediment produced in the United States. Also, 37 percent of all pesticides and 50 percent of all antibiotics used in this country are used by animal agribusinesses.

- Thirty percent of the earth's land surface that is now used for livestock was once wildlife habitat.

- Sixty to seventy percent of the world's fish catch goes to feed livestock.

- CAFO antibiotic use adds an estimated $1.5 billion a year to public health costs.

- It takes 2,000 pounds of grain to produce enough meat and other livestock products to feed a person for a year. However, if that person ate the grain directly, rather than via animal products, it would take only 400 pounds of grain.

- The methane produced by cattle and their manure has a global-warming effect equivalent to that of 33 million automobiles.

- Greenhouse gases produced by livestock constitute 37 percent of all methane, 65 percent of nitrous oxide, and 64 percent of ammonia in the atmosphere.

Democracy or Meatocracy?

Bureaucracy helps render genocide unreal.
It ... diminishes the emotional and intellectual tones
associated with the killing. ... There is only a flow of
events to which most people ... come to say yes. ...
Mass murder is everywhere but at the same time ... nowhere.
—Robert Jay Lifton, **The Nazi Doctors**

Violent ideologies speak their own language; core concepts are translated to maintain the system while appearing to support the people. Under carnism, for instance, democracy has become defined as having the freedom to choose among products that sicken our bodies and pollute our planet, rather than the freedom to eat our food and breathe our air without the risk of being poisoned. But violent ideologies are inherently undemocratic, as they rely on deception, secrecy, concentrated power, and coercion—all practices that are incompatible with a free society. While the larger system, or nation, may appear democratic, the violent system within it is not. This is one reason we don't recognize violent ideologies that exist within seemingly democratic systems; we simply aren't thinking to look for them.

In a democratic society, a central role of government is to create and implement policies and legislation that are in the best interest of its citizens. We therefore assume that the food that makes it to our plates isn't going to sicken or kill us. We assume this because we believe that those in our government work for us, the people who pay their salary; we assume the democratic process buffers us from those who might harm us.

However, when power is sufficiently concentrated within an industry, democracy becomes corrupted. Such is the case with meat. Animal agribusiness is a $125 billion industry controlled by just a handful of corporations. These corporations are so powerful because they have become increasingly consolidated, buying out all related businesses, including agro-chemical and seed companies, which produce pesticides, fertilizer, seeds, and other products; processing companies that buy and process livestock; food manufacturers that process the meat into specific products such as frozen entrees; food retailers, including supermarkets and restaurant chains; transportation systems, including railroads and shipping lines; pharmaceuticals; farm equipment such as

tractors and irrigators; and even financial management plans. Econo-
mists warn that when any industry has a concentration ratio that runs
upwards of four companies controlling over 40 percent of the market
(called CR4), competitiveness declines and serious issues, notably in
the area of consumer protection, arise; the conglomerates are able to
set prices and determine, for instance, food quality. The meat industry
far exceeds CR4; for example, four beef packing companies control
83.5 percent of the beef market.[72] The power of animal agribusiness is
such that the industry has become intertwined with government, blurring the boundary between private interests and public service.

One process that has enabled the intertwining of the public and
private sectors is the "revolving door" through which corporate executives and governmental officers exchange positions and strengthen
networks. For instance, in 2004 both the current and former heads
of the Grain Inspection, Packers and Stockyards Administration
(GIPSA)—a division of the USDA that facilitates the marketing of
livestock and other agricultural products—had worked with trade
groups in the meatpacking industry.[73] And the then–USDA secretary Ann Veneman and other high-ranking officials had close former connections to agribusiness, especially in those industries they
were supposed to oversee: Dale Moore, Veneman's chief of staff, was
executive director for legislative affairs of the trade association National Cattlemen's Beef Association (NCBA); James Moseley, deputy
secretary, co-owned a CAFO; and Mary Waters, assistant secretary
for congressional relations, was legislative counsel and senior director for ConAgra, one of the nation's leading meat corporations.[74]

Another reason for such public-private overlap is the massive political funding and lobbying efforts on behalf of the meat industry. For
example, in 2008 the livestock industry contributed over $8 million
to congressional candidates. (And often, much of the contributions
from agribusiness giants end up going to those on the House and

Senate agriculture committees.)[75] Lobbyists promote their client's agenda to legislators. The success of lobbyists' efforts depends largely on the strength of their relationship with government officials; the more lobbyists can afford to provide politicians with niceties ranging from extravagant vacations to exclusive career opportunities, the stronger their relationship with those they seek to influence.

Put simply, the meat industry can influence legislation to benefit itself, at great cost to us. Consider, for example, how the law requires that animal agribusinesses clean up at least some of the mess they've made after dumping their wastes—and yet it doesn't stipulate that these multibillion-dollar corporations cover the bill for their own cleanup. The Environmental Quality Incentives Program (EQIP), a federal program that was ostensibly created to help improve the environmental quality and practices of farmlands and farmers, subsidizes the cleanup. EQIP has doled out $9 billion to help agricultural corporations neutralize the wastes they've dumped.[76] In other words, we help foot the bill for the damage done by corporations such as ConAgra, whose CEO earned $10.8 million in fiscal year 2007.[77] Animal agribusiness subsidies have been criticized by those across the political spectrum as one of the most egregious corporate welfare programs in the history of the United States.

Consider, too, the USDA's gross mismanagement of the deadly *E. coli* public health threat in 2002. Children who had eaten contaminated hamburgers became infected with the bacteria. Symptoms of *E. coli* infection include fever, vomiting, defecating blood, bruising, bleeding from the nose and mouth, swelling of the face and hands, high blood pressure, and, eventually, renal failure. Both ConAgra—the company that had sold the beef—and the USDA had allegedly known the meat was contaminated, yet took no action until two years later, when a full-blown outbreak forced the recall of 19 million pounds of meat that had already been released into the nation's food supply.[78]

If your child were one of those who had become ill from eating contaminated beef, you might want to warn others about the safety of their meat. And this course of action might be effective—as long as you don't make the mistake Oprah Winfrey did and reach too many people at once. In 1996, Winfrey was sued for over $10 million by a group of Texas beef producers for libeling beef. At the height of the mad cow scare in Britain, when twenty people had died from eating what was believed to be tainted beef, Winfrey claimed, on the air, that she would not eat another burger. Under the "food libel laws," legislation that predated the Winfrey case and has been backed by agricultural corporations, it is *illegal* to criticize certain foods without producing "reasonable" scientific evidence. So you might find that, when it comes to speaking out about the meat industry, some restrictions may apply—most notably those on your First Amendment rights.

When animal agribusinesses have become so powerful that they are not only above the law, but also of the law—shaping rather than respecting legislation—we can safely say our democracy has become a meatocracy.

Surgeon General's Warning: Eating Animal Products May Be Hazardous to Your Health

If you walked into your local convenience store and bought a package of cigars, you would notice that it carries a label warning of the potential dangers of cigar smoke. Yet research suggests that cigar smoking poses a hazard only to moderate to heavy cigar smokers, who comprise less than 1 percent of the adult population. More than 97 percent of American adults, however, eat animal foods, and despite much research demonstrating the connection between the consumption of animal products and disease, we are not warned of these dangers.

The vast majority, perhaps 80 to 90 percent of all cancers, cardiovascular diseases, and other forms of degenerative illness can be prevented, at least until very old age, simply by adopting a plant-based [vegetarian] diet.
—T. Colin Campbell, Ph.D., M.S., Professor Emeritus of Nutritional Biochemistry at Cornell University and best-selling author of **The China Study,** *the most comprehensive study of health and nutrition conducted to date*

But let's imagine that you walked into that same convenience store to buy a hot dog. Now imagine that the U.S. Department of Public Health had reviewed studies from the Harvard School of Public Health and other major research institutions and saw fit to include a warning label on animal foods. The label might read something like this:

Surgeon General's Warning: Eating Meat Can Increase Your Risk of Dying from Heart Disease by 50 Percent.[79] **Surgeon General's Warning:** Eating Meat Can Increase Your Risk of Developing Colon Cancer by 300 Percent and Significantly Increase Your Risk of Developing Certain Other Cancers.[80] **Surgeon General's Warning:** Daily Meat Consumption Can Triple Your Risk of Prostate Enlargement and Regular Milk Consumption Doubles Your Risk.[81] **Surgeon General's Warning:** The Animal That Became Your Meat May Have Been Fed Euthanized Cats and Dogs; Rendered Feathers, Hooves, Hair, Skin, Blood, and Intestines; Road Kill; Animal Manure; Plastic Pellets That Were Harvested from Dead Cows' Rumen; and Carcasses from Animals of Their Own Species. **Surgeon General's Warning:**

This Product May Contain Dangerous Levels of Pesticides, Arsenic, Antibiotics, and Hormones. **Surgeon General's Warning:** This Product May Contain Microbial Organisms That Could Lead to Illness or Death. **Surgeon General's Warning:** Production of This Food Has Contributed to Serious Environmental Degradation, Animal Cruelty, and Human Rights Violations. **Surgeon General's Warning:** There Is Shit in Your Meat.

But, of course, meat products come with no such warnings, despite the fact that these foods are consumed by hundreds of millions of people on a regular basis. Violent ideologies follow their own logic, the logic that sustains the system—a convoluted logic that unravels when it, itself, is labeled.

As we've discussed, the most notable characteristic of all violent ideologies is invisibility, both symbolic (by not being named) and literal (by keeping the violence out of sight). I have, therefore, attempted to illuminate the hidden aspects of carnism, so that you might understand the truth about the production of animal foods and why the system works so diligently to remain unseen.

Yet invisibility can only protect us so much. Hints of the truth surround us: "cruelty-free" veggie burgers at the grocery store; the resilient vein in the drumstick that's suddenly reminiscent of a living chicken; snapshots of meatpacking plants that occasionally make the news; vegetarian guests at dinner parties; dead piglets hanging in the windows of Chinatown markets; the hog on a spit at the company barbecue; and an endless supply of dead animals in the form of meat. So when invisibility inevitably falters, we need a backup, something to protect us from the truth and to help us quickly recover should we suddenly begin to catch on to the disturbing reality of carnism. We must replace the *reality* of meat with the *mythology* of meat.

CHAPTER 5

THE MYTHOLOGY OF MEAT:
JUSTIFYING CARNISM

If we believe absurdities, we shall commit atrocities.
—*Voltaire*

Unthinking respect for authority
is the greatest enemy of truth.
—*Albert Einstein*

It is a sunny afternoon, and the petting zoo outside the local grocery store has drawn its usual crowd. Children and their parents are pressed up against the wooden fence, some leaning over it with arms outstretched. I take out one of the carrots I brought for this occasion and offer it to a piglet, hoping to lure it close enough for me to pet it. For some reason, I always feel an urge to physically connect with the animals. It seems almost instinctive, the desire to touch, to pet them.

And I am not alone. I watch as wide-eyed children shriek with delight when a piglet accepts one of their offerings and they get a chance to steal a fleeting stroke of its cheek or head. I see the adults laugh affectionately as the baby animal unselfconsciously gobbles down its food, unfazed by the eager little hands around it. I notice the attention the lone cow is getting, beckoned from all sides. When she chooses, for no apparent reason, my fistful of grass, I am warmed. I pet her velvety nose as others cluster around me to touch her head and neck.

Even the chickens elicit interest and amusement. Children squat down to toss bread crumbs through the openings in the fence, smiling openmouthed as the birds peck at the ground and occasionally pause with heads cocked to observe the crowd. Not surprisingly, the onlookers comment on how adorable the fuzzy chicks are as they peep and hop around with no apparent focus.

It is a sight to behold. Children giggle and clap, mothers and fathers smile fondly, and everyone seems determined to touch and be touched by the pigs, cows, and chickens. Yet these people, who feel so deeply compelled to make contact with the animals, and who as children may have wept when they read *Charlotte's Web* and fallen asleep hugging their stuffed pigs or calves—these same people will soon leave the grocery store with bags containing beef, ham, and chicken. These people, who would undoubtedly rush to the aid of one of the barnyard animals were it suffering, are somehow not *outraged* that ten billion of them are suffering needlessly every year, within the confines of an industry that is left entirely unaccountable for its actions.

Where has our empathy gone?

The Three Ns of Justification

In order to consume the meat of the very species we had caressed but minutes before, we must believe so fully in the justness of eating animals that we are spared the consciousness of what we are doing. To this end, we are taught to accept a series of myths that maintain the carnistic system and to ignore the inconsistencies in the stories we tell ourselves. Violent ideologies rely on promoting fiction as fact and discouraging any critical thinking that threatens to expose this truth.

There is a vast mythology surrounding meat, but all the myths are in one way or another related to what I refer to as the Three Ns of Justification: eating meat is *normal, natural,* and *necessary.* The Three Ns have been invoked to justify all exploitative systems, from African slavery to the Nazi Holocaust. When an ideology is in its prime, these myths rarely come under scrutiny. However, when the system finally collapses, the Three Ns are recognized as ludicrous. Consider, for instance, the following justifications for why women were denied the right to vote in the United States: male-only voting was "designed by our forefathers"; if women were to vote, it would "cause irreparable damage . . . to the state" and "disaster and ruin would take over the nation."

The Three Ns are so ingrained in our social consciousness that they guide our actions without our even having to think about them. They think for us. We have internalized them so fully that we often live in accordance with their tenets as though they were universal truths rather than widely held opinions. It's like driving a car— once you've learned to do it, you no longer need to think about every action. But these justifications do more than just direct our actions. They alleviate the moral discomfort we might otherwise feel when eating meat; if we have a good excuse for our behaviors, we feel less guilty about them. The Three Ns essentially act as mental and emotional blinders, masking the discrepancies in our beliefs and behaviors toward animals and explaining them away if we do happen to catch on.

Meet the Mythmakers

Despite the falsehoods that weave our psychological and emotional safety net, it takes energy to suppress the truth. It takes an ongoing effort to remain blind to what is right in front of us, to stay oblivious to the glaring inconsistencies, and to keep our authentic feelings from surfacing. So, though we have become adept at ignoring the part of us that knows the truth, we must be continually coached to maintain the disconnection between our awareness and our empathy.

Enter the mythmakers. The mythmakers occupy every sector of society, ensuring that no matter where we turn, the information we are given reinforces the Three Ns. The mythmakers are the institutions that form the pillars of the system, and the people who represent them. When a system is entrenched, it is supported by every major institution in society, from medicine to education; chances are, your doctors and teachers didn't encourage you to question whether meat is normal, natural, and necessary. Nor did your parents, pastor, or elected officials. Who better to influence us than the establishments and professionals in whom we have learned to place our trust? Who better to convince us than those in positions of authority?

Indeed, professionals play a key role in sustaining violent ideologies. One way they do this is by modeling the tenets of the ideology. In the case of carnism, professionals model attitudes and practices toward animals with their policies and recommendations—and their own behaviors. Consider, for instance, the endorsement of the American Veterinary Medical Association (AVMA)—the "voice of the veterinary community"—of gestation crates, two-foot-wide stalls in which sows are confined during pregnancy. As I mentioned in chapter 3, these enclosures are considered so inhumane they've been banned in a number of nations and states, and even corporations such as Mc-Donalds oppose them. Consider, too, that many veterinarians eat and wear animals.

Professionals also model the tenets of carnism by acting as "voices of reason," as "rational moderates"[82] in the debate about how animals should be treated. These people have been called "socialized critics"[83] because they lend credibility to the system by supporting the overall ideology while opposing some of its mores. The rational moderate stance of professionals makes those who challenge the system appear to be "irrational extremists" by contrast. A common example of rational moderates is veterinarians who oppose certain factory-farming practices but regularly eat meat.

Another way professionals help sustain a violent ideology is by pathologizing or thwarting those who don't support it, as with psychologists who assume that a young woman's refusal to eat meat is symptomatic of an eating disorder or doctors who warn of the dangers of a meat-free diet despite much evidence to the contrary. However, though professional support is essential for maintaining carnism, in general, professionals themselves don't consciously bolster the ideology. Professionals are simply people doing their jobs; they are people who were raised within the system and therefore, like the rest of us, see the world through the lens of carnism.

But not all mythmakers are unaware of the stories they spin. Another group of mythmakers, the animal agribusinesses and their executives, actively sustains the myths of meat by influencing the institutions and professionals that in turn impact policy and opinion. Consider, for instance, the partnership between the American Dietetic Association (ADA) and the National Dairy Council. The ADA is the nation's leading organization of nutritionists, and it is also the governing body that oversees the accreditation of universities that offer degrees in dietetics; all registered dietitians are required to have graduated from an ADA-accredited institution. The National Dairy Council is one of the ADA's leading "corporate sponsors." According to the ADA, their Corporate Sponsorship Program helps corporations have "access to key influencers, thought leaders and decision-makers in the food and nutrition marketplace." And, the ADA says, the sponsor "can leverage benefits to achieve marketing objectives . . . gain access to food and nutrition leaders who influence and make critical purchasing decisions . . . [and] build brand relevance with [the ADA's] highly-desirable target audience."[84] In other words, institutional power holders such as the National Dairy Council "sponsor" professional institutions like the ADA—which may help to explain, for instance, the official recommended daily allowance of three cups of milk, despite evidence linking dairy consumption with an increased risk of cardiovascular disease, various cancers, and diabetes.

However, though the mythmakers distort the truth, their primary role lies not in creating myths, but in making sure the existing ones continue to thrive. So they function largely as *emissaries* of the myths. Many of our myths of meat have been inherited, passed down through the generations; because systems are greater than the sum of their parts, they don't die a natural death, but live on indefinitely. Systems are like beehives: even though individual bees die, the swarm persists. The mythmakers thus recycle the myths of meat, amending them when necessary to fit the current trend.

Questioning Authority

Stanley Milgram's now-classic study on obedience to authority demonstrates just how vulnerable we are to authority figures. In the early 1960s, Milgram recruited forty male subjects and told them that they would act as "teachers" in an experiment on the effects of punishment on learning. When each subject arrived, he was paired with another subject, a "learner." Unbeknownst to the teachers, the learners were actually Milgram's accomplices. The pair was taken to a room where the learner was strapped to a chair and hooked up to what appeared to be electrodes. The men were told that the teacher was to call out word pairs for the learner to memorize, and if the learner didn't memorize them correctly, he'd be shocked by the teacher. With each subsequent mistake, the shock would increase in intensity. The teacher was taken to another room, which had an electric console that supposedly connected to the electrodes on the learner. On the console the shock voltages ranged from 15 to 450, and next to the highest voltage a sign read "Danger—Severe Shock."

In the beginning stages of the experiment, the learner remembered the word pairs accurately. But eventually, he started making mistakes. With the first few shocks, the learner groaned and made sounds of discomfort. By 150 volts, the learner was complaining that he was in pain and insisted on being released from the experiment. At 285 volts, the learner screamed in agony. All during this time, Milgram was instructing the teacher to continue. And most of the teachers did—a staggering thirty-four of the forty subjects shocked the learner even after he had demanded to be released, and twenty-six of those thirty-four continued the shocks all the way up to 450 volts. The teachers were clearly in distress, sweating, holding their heads, complaining—and yet they continued. Milgram repeated his experiment again and again, with different groups and in different contexts, and each time the results were the same. He concluded that *obedience to authority overrides one's conscience.*

Milgram's conclusion is chilling, but not surprising. History is replete with examples of atrocities ranging from unjust wars to genocides, all of which were made possible by millions of people who followed the dictates of their leaders, people whose consciences had been deactivated by those in positions of authority.

Milgram did, however, find that there are two mitigating factors in one's obedience to authority: the ability to question the legitimacy of the authority figure and the distance one has from the figure. For instance, when Milgram had an "ordinary man" (one who seemed not to be a researcher) give the commands to administer shocks, obedience dropped by two-thirds; subjects saw the researcher more as an equal than an authority. And when the researcher wasn't in the room with the teacher, obedience also dropped by two-thirds; the teachers would cheat.

Milgram believes that we act against our conscience because when a command comes from someone we perceive to be a legitimate authority, we don't see ourselves as fully responsible for our actions. And the closer in proximity this person is to us—whether it's a doctor giving us dietary advice or a celebrity on the television set in our living room telling us that "milk does a body good"—the more likely their authority will override our own. Until we learn to question external authority and acknowledge our own, internal authority, we will follow the decrees of those who maintain the status quo.

The Official Seal of Approval: Legitimation

The [Nazi] destruction process required the cooperation of every sector of German society. The bureaucrats drew up the definitions and decrees; the churches gave evidence of Aryan descent; the postal authorities carried the messages of deportation; business corporations dismissed their Jewish employees and took over ... properties; the railroads carried the victims to their place of execution ... the operation required and received the participation of every major social, political and religious institution of the German Reich.
—Richard Rubenstein, theologian

The practical goal of the myths is to *legitimize* the system. When an ideology is legitimized, its tenets are sanctioned by all social institutions and the Three Ns are disseminated through all social channels. Acting in accordance with the ideology is lawful, and it is considered reasonable and ethical. Consequently, the tenets of competing ideologies are viewed as *il*legitimate, which is why, for instance, vegetarians cannot press charges against agribusiness owners for the slaughtering of animals.

Though all institutions help legitimize the ideology, two in particular play a critical role: the legal system and the news media. Writing the tenets of an ideology into law forces conformity to the system. Consider, for instance, how the legal status of animals ensures continued meat production. Under U.S. law, one can be either a legal *person* or legal *property*. A legal person is entitled to basic rights, most notably the right to live free from being physically violated by another. In contrast, legal property has no rights; only the legal person who owns the property has rights, which is why, for instance, you can sue someone who damages your car, but the car itself cannot press charges. Today, all humans are legal persons (though the Constitution originally classified slaves as three-fifths persons, two-fifths property), and all animals are legal property—and person-owners have the right to do what they will with their private property, with few exceptions. So animals are bought and sold, eaten and worn—and their bodies are used in such a wide variety of products that it's virtually impossible not to conform to the system. Animal by-products can be found in such unexpected commodities as tennis balls, wallpaper, adhesive bandages, and film.

The news media, our primary source of information, bolster carnism by acting as a direct channel from the ideology to the consumer. When it comes to carnism, the media fail to challenge the system and support carnistic defenses: they maintain the invisibility of the system and reinforce the justifications for eating meat.

One way the media maintain carnistic invisibility is through *omission*. The ten billion animals that are killed every year for meat and the virulent consequences of contemporary animal agricultural practices remain conspicuously absent from public discourse. How often have you seen media exposés on the violent treatment of farm animals and the corrupt practices of carnistic industry? Compare this with the amount of coverage afforded fluctuating gas prices or Hollywood fashion blunders. Most of us are more outraged over having to pay five cents more for a gallon of gas than over the fact that billions of animals, millions of humans, and the entire ecosystem are systematically exploited by an industry that profits from such gratuitous violence. And most of us know more about what the stars wore to the Oscars than we do about the animals we eat.

The media also maintain the invisibility of the system through *prohibition,* through actively preventing anticarnist information from reaching consumers. For instance, in 2004, CBS turned down $2 million from the animal rights group People for the Ethical Treatment of Animals (PETA), which wanted to air an antimeat advertisement during the Super Bowl. The network claimed the station didn't air "advocacy advertisements." However, CBS did run an antismoking advertisement during the game, and the station regularly airs commercials that promote meat consumption.

Sometimes, however, meat production does get media attention. But when this happens, the issue is usually presented as if it were an aberration rather than the norm. For example, in the exposé of a meatpacking plant in which downed animals had been processed and included in schoolchildren's meat that we discussed in chapter 3, there was no mention of the fact that the facility had been *randomly* targeted by Humane Society of the United States investigators, nor was there discussion of the potential prevalence of this practice among carnistic corporations. Thus, public outrage was directed toward only a single company, and the system itself remained unchallenged.

Indeed, the system remains unchallenged whenever the media present the tenets of carnism as fact rather than opinion, and the proponents of carnism as objective truth tellers rather than biased mythmakers. Major media venues, for instance, regularly feature segments on how to celebrate holidays that are organized around meat consumption, explaining how to prepare a traditional Thanksgiving turkey or host a Fourth of July cookout. And the doctors and nutritionists who appear in the media virtually always advocate carnism, often assuming a "reasonable moderate" stance by, for example, recommending that viewers replace fatty meats with leaner meats.

The news media deliver carnism to our doorstep by informing us not only of "the way things are," but also of the way things ought to be, are meant to be, and have to be. In other words, the news media bring home the Three Ns.

Eating Meat Is Normal

Custom will reconcile people to any atrocity.
—George Bernard Shaw

When we view the tenets of an ideology as normal, it means the ideology has become *normalized,* and its tenets *social norms.* Social norms aren't merely descriptive—describing how the majority of people behave—they are also prescriptive, dictating how we *ought to* behave. Norms are socially constructed. They aren't innate, and they don't come from God (though some of us may have been taught otherwise); they are created and maintained by people, and they serve to keep us in line so the system remains intact.

Norms keep us in line by laying out paths for us to follow and by teaching us how to be so that we fit in. The path of the norm is the path of least resistance; it is the route we take when we're on autopilot and don't even realize we're following a course of action that we haven't consciously chosen. Most people who eat meat have no idea that they're behaving in accordance with the tenets of a system that has defined many of their values, preferences, and behaviors. What they call "free choice" is, in fact, the result of a narrowly constructed set of options that have been chosen for them. They don't realize, for instance, that they have been taught to value human life so far above certain forms of nonhuman life that it seems appropriate for their taste preferences to supersede other species' preference for survival. And by carving out the path of least resistance, norms obscure alternative paths and make it seem as if there is no other way to be; as I mentioned in chapter 2, meat eating is considered a given, not a choice.

Another way norms keep us in line is by rewarding conformity and punishing us if we stray off course. Practically and socially, it is vastly easier to eat meat than not. Meat is readily available, while nonmeat alternatives must be actively sought out and may be hard to come by. For example, many restaurants still have no vegetarian options listed on the menu, and standard vegetarian fare, such as beans and rice, is frequently cooked with lard and chicken broth. And vegetarians often find themselves having to explain their choices, defend their diet, and apologize for inconveniencing others. They are stereotyped as hippies, eating disordered, and sometimes antihuman. They are called hypocrites if they wear leather, purists or extremists if they don't. They must live in a world where they are constantly bombarded by imagery and attitudes that offend their deepest sensibilities. It is easier by far to conform to the carnistic majority than eschew the path of least resistance.

Norms are reflected in everyday behavior, as well as in customs and traditions. When a behavior is customary or traditional, its longevity and role in maintaining the system make it less likely to be questioned and far easier to justify. For instance, for many people, Thanksgiving simply wouldn't be Thanksgiving without a turkey on the table; rarely is the choice of holiday fare questioned.

Eating Meat Is Natural

[Nazism], unlike any other political philosophy
or Party program, is in accord with the
natural history and biology of man.
—Rudolf Ramm, Nazi medical expert

Most of us believe that eating meat is natural because humans have hunted and consumed animals for millennia. And it is true that we have been eating meat as part of an omnivorous diet for at least two million years (though for the majority of this time our diet was still primarily vegetarian). But to be fair, we must acknowledge that infanticide, murder, rape, and cannibalism are at least as old as meat eating, and are therefore arguably as "natural"—and yet we don't invoke the history of these acts as a justification for them. As with other acts of violence, when it comes to eating meat, we must differentiate between *natural* and *justifiable*.

The way "natural" translates to "justifiable" is through the process of *naturalization*. Naturalization is to natural as normalization is to normal. When an ideology is naturalized, its tenets are believed to be in accordance with the laws of nature (and/or the law of God, depending on whether one's belief system is science- or faith-based, or both). Naturalization reflects a belief in the way things are *meant to* be; eating meat is seen as simply following the natural order of things. Naturalization maintains an ideology by providing it with a (bio)logical basis.

Like norms, many naturalized behaviors are constructed, and it should come as no surprise that they're constructed by those who place themselves at the top of the "natural hierarchy." The belief in the biological superiority of certain groups has been used for centuries to justify violence: Africans were "naturally" suited to slavery; Jews were "naturally" evil and would destroy Germany if not eradicated; women were "naturally" designed to be the property of men; animals "naturally" exist to be eaten by humans. Consider, for instance, how we refer to the animals we eat as though nature designed them for this very purpose: we call them "farm" (rather than "farmed") animals, "broiler chickens," "dairy cows," "layer hens," and "veal calves." Even the great logician Aristotle invoked biology and bent logic to suit the norms of his era, when he asserted that males were naturally superior to females and slaves were biologically designed to serve free men. And consider one of the central justifications for carnism, the natural order of the so-called food chain. Humans supposedly reside at the "top" of the food chain—yet a chain, by definition, doesn't have a top, and if it did, it would be inhabited by carnivores, not omnivores.

The key disciplines that support naturalization are history, religion, and science. History presents us with a selective historical focus and "facts" that prove the ideology has always existed. The historical lens *eternalizes* the ideology, making it seem as if it always has been, and therefore always will be, the way things are. Religion upholds the ideology as divinely ordained, and science provides the ideology with a biological basis. The importance of religion and science in naturalizing an ideology helps to explain why spirituality and intelligence have been popular criteria by which a group defines itself as naturally superior. For instance, before animal experimentation was a common scientific practice, the mathematician and philosopher René Descartes nailed the paws of his wife's dog to a board in order to dissect it alive and prove that, unlike humans but like other animals, the dog was a soulless "machine" whose cries of pain were no different from the springs and wheels of a clock automatically reacting when dismantled. And Charles Darwin argued that because males were supposedly born with a greater capacity for reason than females, over the course of evolution men have become superior to women. In short, naturalization makes the ideology historically, divinely, and biologically irrefutable.

Eating Meat Is Necessary

We of the South will not, cannot, surrender our institutions.
To maintain the existing relations between the two races
[whites and blacks] ... is indispensable to
the peace and happiness of both.
—*John. C. Calhoun, former Vice President of the United States*

The belief that eating meat is necessary is closely connected to the belief that eating meat is natural; if meat eating is a biological imperative, then it is a necessity for the survival of the (human) species. And, as with all violent ideologies, this belief reflects the core paradox of the system: killing is necessary for the greater good; the survival of one group depends on the killing of another.[85] The belief that eating meat is necessary makes the system seem inevitable—if we cannot exist without meat, then abolishing carnism is akin to suicide. Though we know that it's possible to survive without eating meat, the system proceeds as if this myth were true; it is an implicit assumption that is typically only revealed when challenged.

A related myth is that meat is necessary for our health. This myth, too, persists in the face of overwhelming evidence to the contrary. If anything, research suggests that eating meat is detrimental to health, as meat consumption has been connected with the development of some of the major diseases of the modern industrialized world.

The Protein Myth

But where do you get your protein?

This is often the first response a vegetarian hears after disclosing his or her dietary orientation. In fact, this question is so common as to be a running joke among vegetarians across the nation. I use the term "joke" because the question reflects one of, if not the, most common and unrealistic myths about carnism: that meat is a necessary source of protein. Vegetarians refer to this misconception as the Protein Myth.

The fear of becoming protein deficient is especially common among men, as (animal) protein has traditionally been associated with building muscle and strength. Meat has long been a symbol of masculinity, as it represents power, might, and virility; conversely, plant-based foods have been feminized, often representing passivity and weakness (consider the meaning of the phrases "couch potato" and "veg out"). There is a growing body of literature examining how masculinity has been constructed—to the detriment of individuals and society—largely around dominance, control, and violence. It should come as no surprise, then, that consuming (and sometimes killing) animals has been a central feature of manhood. [86]

Like other myths of meat, the Protein Myth exists in the face of longstanding, widespread, and substantial evidence to the contrary; it acts to justify continued meat consumption and maintain the carnistic paradigm. But it is, indeed, a myth. Here's what doctors have to say:

> In the early 1900s, Americans were told to eat well over 100 grams of protein a day. And as recently as the 1950s, health-conscious people were encouraged to boost their protein intake. Today . . . Americans tend to take in twice the amount of protein they need. . . . Excess protein has been linked with osteoporosis, kidney disease, calcium stones in the urinary tract, and some cancers.
>
> People build muscle and other body proteins from amino acids, which come from the proteins they eat. A varied diet of beans, lentils, grains, and vegetables contains all of the essential amino acids. It was once thought that various plant foods had to be eaten together to get their full protein value, but current research suggests this is not the case.
>
> To consume a diet that contains enough, but not too much, protein, [one can] simply replace animal products with grains, vegetables, legumes (peas, beans, and lentils), and fruits. As long as one is eating a variety of plant foods in sufficient quantity to maintain one's weight, the body gets plenty of protein.[87]

One particularly striking myth of necessity is the belief that we must continue to eat meat because if we were to stop now, the world would be overrun by pigs, chickens, and cows. What, we wonder, would we do with all the animals? Of course, if we stopped eating meat, we'd stop producing the animals that become our meat in the first place, so we'd be safe from being overwhelmed by a burgeoning population of farmed animals. And there is a myth within this myth, a paradox that is central to all violent ideologies—that killing must continue in order to justify all the killing already done.[88] Once the momentum of the violence has reached a certain point, reversing it seems impossible.

Another myth of necessity is that killing is an economic imperative. While an economic motive *has* driven many violent ideologies—the economy of the New World was largely buttressed by slavery, and the plundering of gold and other assets as well as the unpaid labor of Nazi victims financed the German war machine—that doesn't mean the economy would collapse were the killing to cease. It is far more likely that the economic status quo would break down; the carnistic-corporate power structure, rather than the citizenry, would suffer were carnism abolished.

Even were the economy dependent on carnism, one must wonder whether this dependence would justify the continued violence. For most people, it would not. History shows us again and again that, when people become aware of violent ideologies, they demand change. It is for this reason that the atrocities of carnism must remain hidden and the myths of carnism must remain intact—that we must believe we are informed consumers and free agents acting within a democratic system, exercising our own free will.

The Myth of Free Will

Violent ideologies require willing participants, and most Americans would not willingly harm animals. Thus, people must be coerced into supporting the system. However, coercion is effective only as long as it remains undetected. We must believe we are acting entirely of our own volition when we purchase and consume the bodies of animals; we must believe in the Myth of Free Will.

Of course, nobody's putting a gun to our heads when we eat meat, but they don't have to. From the moment we were weaned, we were eating animals. Did you freely choose to eat your Gerber Turkey and Rice Dinner? How about when you were a child, eating your Mc-Donald's Happy Meal? And did you question your parents and teachers and doctors when they told you meat made you strong? Did you ever look at the meatballs atop your pasta and wonder where they really came from? If so, did the people around you encourage you to close the gap in your consciousness, or did they quickly restore your numbing and reassure you of the virtues of meat?

Chances are, the pattern by which you have related to meat started before you were old enough to talk and has continued uninterrupted throughout your life. And it is in this flow of uninterrupted behavior that we may see how carnism washes over free will. Patterns of thought and behavior, established long before we were able to act as free agents, become woven into the fabric of our psyche, guiding our choices like an invisible hand. And if something should interrupt our habitual way of relating to meat—if, for instance, we catch a glimpse of the slaughter process—the elaborate network that makes up the defensive structure of carnism pulls us swiftly back in. *Carnism blocks interruptions in consciousness.*

It is impossible to exercise free will as long as we are operating from within the system. Free will requires consciousness, and our pervasive and deep-seated patterns of thought are unconscious; they are outside of our awareness and therefore outside of our control. While we remain in the system, we see the world through the eyes of carnism. And as long as we look through eyes other than our own, we will be living in accordance with a truth that is not of our own choosing. We must step outside the system to find our lost empathy and make choices that reflect what we truly feel and believe, rather than what we've been taught to feel and believe.

CHAPTER 6

THROUGH THE CARNISTIC LOOKING GLASS: INTERNALIZED CARNISM

The greatest enemy of knowledge is not ignorance;
it is the illusion of knowledge.
—Stephen Hawking

Imagine if everything that constitutes your reality—your home, your job, your family, your *life*—were nothing more than an illusion, a virtual reality, fabricated by a computerized matrix that your brain and the brains of all other humans were plugged into. Imagine this matrix uses us as batteries; it siphons off our energy to keep itself alive and keeps us complacent by remaining invisible while generating the illusion of our freedom. Such is the theme of *The Matrix,* a film that resonated so powerfully with millions of viewers that it was heralded as a modern classic. Classics attain their status because they speak to a core human experience. They give voice to truths that have been largely elusive and thus unspoken. *The Matrix* challenges us to question—to question what we see, and how we relate to what we see. It challenges us to be curious about what we think and why we think the way we do. Morpheus, a leading character in the film, explains to the protagonist, Neo:

> The Matrix is everywhere. It is all around us. Even now, in this very room. You can see it when you look out your win-

dow or when you turn on your television. You can feel it when you go to work . . . when you go to church . . . when you pay your taxes. It is the world that has been pulled over your eyes to blind you to the truth . . . [it is] *a prison for your mind.*

Neo's mind was imprisoned by a matrix, a system so entrenched that it had effectively stripped him of the ability to think for himself. And by accepting the illusions of the Matrix as real, Neo helped authenticate the system; he was at once prisoner and captor, victim and perpetrator.

Likewise, the matrix of meat that is carnism compels us to participate in our own coercion, doing the system's job for it: we deny, avoid, and justify carnism. When our minds are imprisoned by carnism, we see the world—and ourselves—through the eyes of the system. As a result, we behave not as we actually are, but as the system would like us to be: we are passive consumers rather than active citizens. The mechanisms of the system have become ingrained into our consciousness. We have *internalized* carnism.

The Cognitive Trio

Carnism distorts reality: Just because we don't see the animals we eat, this doesn't mean they don't exist. Just because the system hasn't been named, this doesn't mean it isn't real. No matter how far they stretch and how deep they run, the myths of meat are not the facts of meat.

Internalized carnism distorts our *perception* of reality: though animals are living beings, we perceive them as living things; though they are individuals, we perceive them as abstractions—as a "bunch" of things; and in the absence of any objective, supporting data, we perceive them as though their appropriateness for human consumption is naturally contingent upon their species. For instance, if, despite the system's best efforts, we happen to catch sight of one of the pigs who is to become our meat, we don't perceive him or her as a sentient being, or as someone who has a distinct personality and preferences. Rather, we perceive the pig's "pigness" (dirtiness, slovenliness, etc.) and his or her "edibility." By perceiving animals in these ways, we employ three defenses that I refer to as the Cognitive Trio.

The Cognitive Trio is comprised of *objectification, deindividualization,* and *dichotomization.* These defenses are actually normal psychological processes that become defensive distortions when used excessively, as they must be in order to keep carnism intact. And, unlike some other defenses, these mechanisms are more internal and less conscious and intentional; they are less about *what* we think than they are about *how* we think. Each defense in the Cognitive Trio has a unique effect on our perception of animals. But the true strength of the trio lies in how the three work in harmony with one another. Like a musical trio, the whole is greater than the sum of its parts.

Objectification: Viewing Animals as Things

The more you see these lambs without any heads on them,
the more you don't think of them as an animal,
but as a product that you're working with.
—Thirty-one-year-old male meat cutter[*]

Objectification is the process of viewing a living being as an inanimate object, a thing. Animals are objectified in a variety of ways, perhaps most notably through language. Objectifying language is a powerful

---

[*]Selected quotes in this chapter are from interviews I conducted for my doctoral dissertation on the psychology of meat.

distancing mechanism. Consider how slaughterhouse workers refer to the animals they're going to kill as the objects they are to become, rather than as the living animals they are: chickens are called *broilers,* pigs are called *rashers,* and bulls are called *beef.* And the USDA refers to cows as *udders* and animals as *units,* while meat industries talk about *replacement boars* or *replacement calves.* Consider, too, our common usage of the phrase *living thing,* and our equally common failure to recognize this phrase as an oxymoron. Carnism needs us to employ such objectifying language; think of how you might feel if, for instance, you referred to the rotisserie chicken in the restaurant window as some*one* rather than some*thing,* or if you called the barnyard turkey *he* or *she* rather than *it.*

Objectification is legitimized not only through language, but also through institutions, legislation, and policies. For example, as we discussed in chapter 5, the law classifies animals as property. When we can buy, sell, trade, or exchange someone as though he or she were a used car—or even parts of a used car—we have literally turned him or her into a piece of live *stock.* By viewing animals as objects, we can treat their bodies accordingly, without the moral discomfort we might otherwise feel.

Deindividualization: Viewing Animals as Abstractions

I don't [think of farmed animals as individuals]. I wouldn't be able to do my job if I got that personal with them. . . . When you say individuals, you mean as a unique person, as a unique thing with its own name and its own characteristics, its own little games it plays? Yeah? Yeah, I'd really rather not know that. I'm sure it has it, but I'd rather not know it.
—Thirty-one-year-old male meat cutter

Deindividualization is the process of viewing individuals only in terms of their group identity and as having the same characteristics as everyone else in the group. Whenever we encounter a group of others, it's natural for us to think of them, at least in part, as a group. The larger the group, the more likely we are to view the whole over its individual parts; when you think of a nation, for example, you probably think of its citizens primarily as members of a group to which you've ascribed a set of shared characteristics. Deindividualization, however, is viewing others *only* as members of a whole; it is the failure to appreciate the individuality of the parts that make up the whole. Such is the case with our perception of the animals we eat.

For instance, as I mentioned previously, when you think of the pigs raised for pork you probably don't think of them as individuals with their own personalities and preferences. Rather, you see them as an *abstraction,* as a group. Like other groups that have been victims of violent ideologies, pigs raised for meat may have numbers rather than names and are considered no different from one another; a pig is a pig and all pigs are the same. But imagine how you would feel if your package of hot dogs included a label with the name, picture, and description of the pig from whom the meat was procured, or if you became acquainted with one of the pigs who was to become your food. Countless students of mine, as well as the carnists and meat cutters I interviewed in my research, have reported that after getting to know an individual "food" animal, they felt unable to consume that particular animal, and some even felt uncomfortable continuing to eat meat from that species. For instance, a thirty-year-old meat cutter told me, "I would have a different outlook on pigs in general if I had a pig as a pet. . . . I would just see my pet every time someone was preparing ribs or something like that."

Negative reactions to the idea of consuming (or preparing the meat of) a familiar animal are common around the world, and they can be quite powerful. For instance, female Indians from the Quito area in Ecuador bond with their chickens just as Americans do with our dogs and cats, and when circumstances force these women to sell their birds for slaughter, they do so with tears and shrieks.[89] And consider the responses of my interviewees when I asked them how they would react to eating a farmed animal they'd become acquainted with. A thirty-five-year-old female carnist explained, "It would feel wrong to eat that [meat]. . . . I mean, it would feel like I murdered it, you know, that I killed it. And for what? You know what I'm saying? I wouldn't even conceive of it. If it's a pet, it's off limits, you know? Once it dies, you bury it; it's sort of like a family member."

This feeling is echoed by a fifty-eight-year-old butcher, who told me, "I'd have to be starving before I'd eat my own pet [pig] . . . [because] once I knew him or her really well I would be offended to have to eat my friend." Yet when I asked why he doesn't feel the same way about the pigs he processes for his job, he responded, "I must class them all as food. If someone was raising him as a pet, that would be different."

One carnist, a thirty-one-year-old male who had raised and killed his own animals in his native country, Zimbabwe, explained, "I would not eat something that I would give a name to. . . . For me, that's like your friend. You are eating an animal that you have a close relationship with."

Another carnist, a twenty-eight-year-old male, said that he would not even have to be personally acquainted with an animal to feel uncomfortable by his or her individuality: "Even, like, some animal in a cage with hundreds of other animals, if you make this connection [that he or she is an individual], then it's kind of on the same parallel as the family pet. How can you kill a family pet? How can you kill a pig that's in a pen with a hundred others?"

Recognizing the individuality of others interrupts the process of deindividualization, making it more difficult to maintain the psychological and emotional distance necessary to harm them.

Numbers and Numbing

Psychologist Paul Slovic examined the relationship between the number of victims in a traumatic situation and witnesses' responses to their suffering. What he found was that the greater the number of victims, the more witnesses blurred, or depersonalized, individuals and the less they tended to care—and this blurring seemed to start at just two victims. Slovic argues that numbers and numbing go hand in hand. What this means is that individual victims, human or non-human, are much more likely to arouse our compassion than are groups of victims.

Consider, for instance, the 2005 incident in which a sparrow flew into a domino competition in the Netherlands, knocking over 23,000 tiles and ending up shot dead: a website was set up as a tribute to the bird, and it attracted tens of thousands of visitors. Or take the 2001 slaughtering of millions of cattle in the United Kingdom that were believed to have been exposed to hoof-and-mouth disease: despite the demands of animal activists to halt the killing, it wasn't until a newspaper printed a photo of a young calf named Phoenix that the government agreed to change its policy. And when author Annie Dillard told her seven-year-old daughter how it was hard for her to imagine that 138,000 people had drowned in Bangladesh, her daughter replied, "No, it's easy. Lots and lots of dots in blue water."

Mother Teresa was all too familiar with the phenomenon of numbers and numbing. "If I look at the mass," she said, "I will never act."

Source: Paul Slovic, "If I Look at the Mass I Will Never Act: Psychic Numbing and Genocide."

Dichotomization:
Viewing Animals in Categories

I don't know, maybe it's easier to [eat] animals that have
been raised just for the purpose of [being eaten] ... where a
squirrel runs around your backyard and then to have it on
your dinner plate is just kind of disturbing.... It's almost
like a division between the animals you see running around
outside—they are safe from people eating [them].
—Twenty-two-year-old female carnist

Dichotomization is the process of mentally putting others into two, often opposing, categories based on our beliefs about them. In and of itself, classifying others into groups is not problematic. As we discussed in chapter 1, creating mental classifications is a natural process that helps us organize information. Dichotomies, however, are not just classifications; they are dualistic, and as such, they create a black-and-white picture of reality. What results is a divvying up of the world into inflexible, value-laden categories that are usually based on little or inaccurate information. Dichotomization thus enables us to separate groups of individuals in our minds and to harbor very different emotions toward them.

When it comes to meat, the two main categories we have for animals are edible and inedible. And within the edible-inedible dichotomy, we have a number of other category pairs. For example, we eat domesticated rather than wild animals, and herbivores rather than omnivores or carnivores. Most people won't eat animals that they deem intelligent (dolphins), but regularly consume those they believe are not very smart (cows and chickens). Many Americans avoid eating animals that they perceive as cute (rabbits) and instead eat animals that they consider less attractive (turkeys).

Whether the categories into which we've placed animals are accurate is less important than whether we *believe* they're accurate, since the purpose of dichotomization is simply to distance us from the discomfort of eating meat. If we filter our perceptions of animals through categories laden with value judgments, we can, for example, eat our steak while we pet our dog and remain oblivious to the implications of our choices. Dichotomization thus supports justification; it enables us to feel justified eating an animal because, for instance, he or she isn't smart, isn't a pet, isn't cute—isn't edible.

Of course, not all edible animals fall neatly into the categories into which we've placed them. To maintain the carnistic status quo, then, we retain false assumptions about the animals we eat so that we can continue to classify them as edible. Intelligent pigs and chickens are seen as stupid, and handsome turkeys are viewed as ugly.

When pressed to examine our assumptions, however, the arbitrary and irrational nature of dichotomization becomes apparent. Consider, for instance, the confusion expressed by a forty-three-year-old male carnist when I asked him to explain why he doesn't eat lamb:

> [Lambs] are gentle creatures. . . . It's, like, a shame they are killed and we eat them. There are a lot of other things that are also gentle, too, that we eat . . . cows are. We eat them. . . . I don't know how to describe it. It seems like everybody eats cow. It's cheaper. It's affordable, and there are so many of them. But lambs are just different. They're smaller or more cuddly. I don't know. You don't cuddle a cow. Seems like it's okay to eat a cow, but it's not okay to eat a lamb. . . . The difference is weird.

Technology, Distortions, and Distancing

It's easier to think of [farmed animals] in the abstract ....
It makes me think of that quote: "The death of one
person is a tragedy; the death of a group is a statistic."
—*Thirty-three-year-old male carnist*

A discussion about the Cognitive Trio would not be complete without mentioning the role of technology in psychological distortions and distancing. Technology reinforces the trio by enabling us to treat certain animals as objects and abstractions—objects, because they literally become units of production on a disassembly line, and abstractions, because the sheer volume of animals killed for meat inevitably deindividualizes them. Indeed, it is only because of technology that widescale meat production is possible: modern methods enable us to eat billions of animals every year without witnessing a single part of the process by which these animals become our food. This mass production of meat, coupled with our removal from the production process, has made us at once more and less violent toward animals than ever before; we are able to kill more animals but are less desensitized to or comfortable with the fact that we're killing them. Technology has widened the gap between our behaviors and values, and thus enhanced the moral dissonance that the system works so hard to obscure.

But of course, technology often doesn't eradicate all traces of meat production. And when it doesn't, we can find ourselves in the uncomfortable position of recognizing that our meat did, in fact, come from a living being. For instance, a twenty-two-year-old female carnist told me that she didn't eat pork from a market in her town that sold pigs' feet and whole pigs: "I think partially because it reminds me more that you're not just eating—like the piece of meat didn't just fall out of the sky. It's connected to the whole animal . . . instead of just a nicely processed thing that you're eating by itself for dinner. . . . You have to think about it as a whole creature."

Distortions and Disgust

I don't like to eat chicken hearts. . . . I think that it is mainly because [with] the chicken hearts, you can really see that it is a small heart. [If I ate it I'd feel] sick. . . . It's just what we associate the heart to be, and you know, the liver and things like that . . . someone's heart or liver—they're associated with people.
—Twenty-seven-year-old female carnist

By distorting our perceptions of animals, the Cognitive Trio prevents us from *identifying* with them. To identify with others is to see something of yourself in them and to see something of them in yourself—even if the only thing you identify with is the desire to be free from suffering. Identification is a cognitive process, and when we think of animals as objects, abstractions, or items in fixed categories, we diminish this process. And because thoughts affect feelings, the less we identify with others, the less we *empathize* with them. This is what's known in psychology as the similarity principle: we feel more empathy toward those whom we perceive to be more like us. Consider, for example, how you might be more disturbed by the deaths of Americans in a plane crash than by the deaths of other passengers, even if you weren't personally acquainted with anyone on board. Consider, too, the statement of a fifty-eight-year-old butcher I interviewed:

I took my son in [to the butcher shop]—he is eight years old. We had a lamb in there. He likes lamb so he walks in and says, "What's that?"

I go, "That's a lamb."

No big deal, but a couple days later I asked, "Do you want a nice lamb steak?"

"Naw," he said, "I don't think I want lamb. I looked at that animal . . . [and] it was looking back at me."

Just as the degree to which we identify with another determines how much we empathize with him or her, the degree of our empathy determines, in large part, how *disgusted* we feel at the notion of eating him or her.* (Some possible exceptions are animals we mentally classify as disgusting even when they're alive, such as snakes and insects, and certain species we consider "dirty," like rats and pigeons.) The fact that identification and empathy inform disgust may explain why researchers have found that almost all disgusting objects are of animal origin (and those that are not of animal origin often resemble animal products, such as slimy, mucus-like okra). The following diagram represents the correlation between identification, empathy, and disgust:

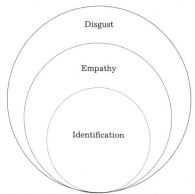

Disgust

Empathy

Identification

*While disgust may be an innate response intended to protect us from ingesting harmful substances, such as feces and rotten vegetation, there is no doubt that it is also a reaction to purely ideational, or psychological, stimuli. Ideational disgust is the focus of this book.

The reason empathy and disgust are so closely connected is because empathy is the foundation of our sense of morality, and disgust is a *moral emotion*. Typically, the more empathy we feel for an animal, the more immoral—and thus disgusted—we feel eating him or her. The connection between morality and disgust is supported by a number of studies that have shown that people feel disgusted by the idea of consuming a product that they find morally offensive, that violates their sense of integrity.[90] Consider the comment of a thirty-four-year-old carnist who regularly enjoys eating meat, but is ethically opposed to eating veal: "Let's just say I came to your house . . . and you told me that I just had veal. I'd probably vomit . . . like I *have to* get that out of my system."

Disgusted by Injustice

A recent study conducted by researchers at the University of Toronto suggests that we may be hardwired to feel disgusted by moral offenses.[91] The researchers attached electrodes to the faces of twenty participants, to record changes in their facial movements. The participants were then subjected to a series of three different conditions: they were given "disgusting" tasting liquids to drink; they looked at photos of disgusting things, such as dirty toilets and injuries; and they were subjected to unfair treatment in a laboratory game they played. The researchers found that in each condition, the subjects' automatic facial movements were the same: they contracted their *levator labii* muscle, which raises the upper lip and wrinkles the nose, indicating a disgust response. The researchers concluded that "moral disgust" may, in fact, be closely linked to the primal, ancient disgust response that protected us from eating rotting or contaminated foods. Other studies have yielded similar results.

Psychological Damage Control:
Disgust and Rationalization

For any number of reasons, we may find ourselves disgusted by the meat of edible animals—meat that isn't supposed to disgust us. In such instances, when disgust breaks through the defenses that keep us numbed, we need a backup defense to act as a safety net; we need to rationalize the irrational.

Rationalization is the defense mechanism by which we provide a rational explanation for something that is not rational. As with other defenses, rationalization serves to keep the system intact. When the carnistic distancing process has been disrupted and disgust arises, we may divert attention from our moral discomfort by blaming our disgust on something other than the fact that we are consuming a living being. For example, when we feel disgusted by meat that reminds us of its animal source, we may attribute our aversion to the texture of the meat or to an imagined health risk. As one interviewee told me, "I don't like eating bacon because . . . it kind of grosses me out. . . . It's saturated with grease. I just can't imagine that being very good for my body. . . . To see that much grease and fat, even if it tasted good, I think it would repulse me." I asked her whether she felt the same way toward french fries, or other greasy foods, and she replied, "It's similar, but there's also something about seeing raw meat when you are cooking. . . . [C]ooking a potato isn't quite as bad, I think. . . . It's that certain connection that [the meat] is a piece of something, not just something that you got out of the ground."

And another interviewee explained, "I won't eat something that is raw or half raw. . . . The sight of blood—I don't like blood, so I sure don't want it running out of my food when I'm eating it." When I asked how the sight of bloody meat made him feel, he responded, "[It's] disgusting. It's not healthy, although I know it's probably more healthy to eat [it] rare than well done."

It is striking how an entire society of rational people can maintain such irrational patterns of thought without catching on to the gaping holes in the logic. And yet this paradox makes sense when understood within the context of carnism: because its modus operandi is to distort rather than report reality, the system is inherently irrational. And because we are looking at the system from within—from within a schema that mirrors it—we have adopted its logic as our own.

Emotional Eating

It is often believed that a culture's avoidance of certain kinds of meat is rational, stemming from the culture's attempt to preserve itself. We assume, for instance, that a culture doesn't advocate eating animals that are unhealthy (think sewer-dwelling rats), useful (like oxen that plow fields), or uneconomical to raise and slaughter (such as carnivorous animals that would be dangerous to handle). However, while in some instances there may be a logical reason for a cultural taboo against consuming a particular type of animal, research suggests that more often, the opposite is true: cultures use explanations such as those above as a way to rationalize their irrational choices of which animals to eat.

In myriad cultures, many species of "edible" animals are perceived as inedible, which strongly suggests that cultural prejudice, rather than logic, determines which animals become classified as food. For example, the Nambikwara Indians of Brazil keep domesticated animals that would be suitable for human consumption, yet treat them instead as pets, interacting with them much as Americans do with dogs and cats; they don't even eat the eggs laid by their hens.[92] Furthermore, there's no reason why Americans shouldn't eat horses, as some French do, or cockroaches, as some Asians do, or pigeons, which are plentiful and consumed in Egypt. Californians could easily harvest the snails that overpopulate their gardens and which are the same species as those served as escargots, but they choose instead to eat only imported snails.[93] And Asian horse people, who have been highly dependent on horses, have no prohibitions against consuming horseflesh. When it comes to deciding which species of animals to eat, it seems that emotion trumps reason.

Picking Out the Dog Meat:
Disgust and Contamination

Disgust has what psychologists call contamination properties. In other words, something disgusting can render anything it comes in contact with disgusting as well. For instance, most of us will not eat soup that a fly has landed in, even if we were able to quickly remove the insect and the surrounding liquid it touched. The remaining soup, with no residual trace of the fly, has become irreparably contaminated. The soup itself wasn't disgusting, but the *idea* that something disgusting—a fly—touched even a small part of it has rendered the soup inedible.

You were first asked to consider the contaminating property of disgust in chapter 1, when you were presented with a scenario in which you were told you had been served dog meat and then were asked whether you would pick the meat out of the stew and just eat the vegetables around it. Chances are, if you had been disgusted by the dog meat, you would also have become disgusted by anything it touched. That is because, unlike *distaste*—disliking the flavor of a product—disgust is often *ideational:* it can be triggered by an idea or belief about a food rather than what that food actually is. The contaminating effect of disgust explains why many vegetarians feel unable to eat food that has been cooked with, or near, meat.*

The Matrix Within the Matrix: The Carnistic Schema

Carnism is a social system, a social matrix. But it is also a psychological system, a system of thought, an *internal* matrix. It is a matrix within the Matrix. And just as the social matrix is set up to maintain the gap in our consciousness, so, too, is the psychological matrix. This psychological matrix is what I call the *carnistic schema.* The carnistic schema is largely comprised of the Cognitive Trio, but it also includes the other defenses and beliefs discussed throughout this book. The carnistic schema is, essentially, the plug that connects us to the broader matrix of carnism.

You may recall from chapter 1 that a schema is the lens through which we view the world, and it serves as a mental classification system that organizes and interprets incoming information. Our carnistic schema dictates which animals are edible and which are inedible, and it determines how—or, more accurately, whether—we feel when we eat meat.

---

*An interesting phenomenon I have observed is that many vegans—"pure" vegetarians who eschew all animal products—tend to be less disgusted by eggs and dairy products than they are by meat. Research on this phenomenon is lacking. However, I suspect that, because it's *possible* to procure eggs and dairy products without violence, these foods are perceived as less morally offensive and thus less disgusting.

Schemas, however, don't only classify information, they also *filter* information; we tend to notice and remember only that which confirms our preexisting assumptions. Psychologists refer to this phenomenon as *confirmation bias*. The carnistic schema selectively allows in information that maintains the gap in our consciousness, and it distorts our perception of information that threatens to close this gap. In other words, the carnistic schema determines what we notice, how we interpret what we notice, and whether we remember what we notice. For instance, during the classroom exercise that I described in chapter 2, in which my students shared their belief that pigs are stupid and disgusting, some of the students later admitted that they had at some point in their lives encountered information discrediting this belief. Yet such information had been quickly forgotten, as their carnistic schema pulled their original view of pigs back into place. Another example of confirmation bias is how the distress people feel upon witnessing footage of animals being slaughtered often "wears off" shortly thereafter.

Tolstoy Syndrome

The phenomenon psychologists refer to as "confirmation bias" has also been called Tolstoy syndrome, after the Russian author who wrote of our tendency to be blinded by our beliefs. As Tolstoy said:

> I know that most men, including those at ease with problems of the greatest complexity, can seldom accept the simplest and most obvious truth if it . . . would oblige them to admit the falsity of conclusions which they have . . . woven, thread by thread, into the fabrics of their life.

The carnistic schema, which twists information so that nonsense seems to make perfect sense, also explains why we fail to see the absurdities of the system. Consider, for instance, advertising campaigns in which a pig dances joyfully over the fire pit where he or she is to be barbecued, or chickens wear aprons while beseeching the viewer to eat them. And consider the Veterinarian's Oath of the American Veterinary Medical Association, "I solemnly swear to use my . . . skills for the . . . relief of animal suffering," in light of the fact that the vast majority of veterinarians eat animals simply because they like the way meat tastes. Or think about how people won't replace their hamburgers with veggie burgers, even if the flavor is identical, because they claim that, if they try hard enough, they can detect a subtle difference in texture. Only when we deconstruct the carnistic schema can we see the absurdity of placing our preference for a flawless re-creation of a textural norm over the lives and deaths of billions of others.

This Way Out: The Crack in the Carnistic Matrix

The carnistic system is riddled with absurdities, inconsistencies, and paradox. It is fortified by a complex network of defenses that make it possible for us to believe without questioning, to know without thinking, and to act without feeling. It is a coercive system that has cultivated in us an elaborate routine of mental gymnastics that keep us from being grounded in our truth. Thus, one cannot help but wonder: *Why all the acrobatics?* Why must the system go to such lengths to keep itself intact?

The answer is simple. Because we care about animals, and we care about the truth. And because the system depends on our not caring, and the system is built on deception. Carnism is a house of cards, a fractured and fragmented system that needs a strong fortress to protect itself from its very own proponents—us.

And like the cinematic Matrix, the matrix of carnism can only imprison our minds and hearts as long as we guard our own cells, as long as we are willing participants. It can only block the truth as long as we can tolerate living a lie. As Morpheus explained to Neo:

> I see it in your eyes. You have the look of a man who accepts what he sees because he is expecting to wake up. . . . Let me tell you why you're here. You're here because you know something. What you know you can't explain, but you feel it. You've felt it your entire life, that there's something wrong with the world. You don't know what it is, but it's there, like a splinter in your mind. . . . I'm trying to free your mind, Neo. But I can only show you the door. You're the one who has to walk through it.

Like Neo, you're here, reading this book, because you've known something is wrong with the world. You are ready to step outside of the carnistic matrix and reclaim the empathy the system has worked so hard to protect you from, the very empathy that leads to the door of carnism—the empathy that will help you walk *through* that door to create a more humane society.

CHAPTER 7

BEARING WITNESS:
FROM CARNISM TO COMPASSION

In a dark time, the eye begins to see.
—*Theodore Roethke*

Our grandchildren will ask us one day: Where were you during the Holocaust of the animals? What did you do against these horrifying crimes? We won't be able to offer the same excuse for the second time, that we didn't know.
—*Helmut Kaplan*

In November 1995, Emily the cow stood in a lineup of bovines in a New England slaughterhouse, awaiting her turn to pass through the swinging doors to the kill floor. Perhaps it was the smell of blood, or the fact that those who had gone before her didn't return, but Emily suddenly charged out of the line, sprinted toward the five-foot-high fence that corralled the grounds, and hefted her 1,500-pound body over the top. She fled through the woods and eluded the incredulous workers who chased after her.

For forty frigid days and nights, Emily hid from her pursuers in the wooded areas of Hopkinton, Massachusetts, a small rural town in the heart of New England. And though A. Arena & Sons, the owners of the slaughterhouse from which Emily escaped, were determined to capture her, the locals were determined to aid her in her flight to freedom. Farmers left out bales of hay for her; residents deliberately misled police by giving false information about her location.

Lewis and Megan Randa, founders of the nearby Peace Abbey, a spiritual and educational center for nonviolent living, learned of Emily's plight. The Randas offered to buy Emily from A. Arena & Sons. They hoped that Emily could live out her life in the small animal sanctuary on their grounds. The owner of the slaughterhouse, Frank Arena, was moved by Emily's story and agreed to sell the $500 cow for just $1. This unexpected act of benevolence was followed by another: film producer Ellen Little, who bought the rights to Emily's story for a sum that covered the cow's care for the rest of her life, donated an extra $10,000 to build Emily a new barn and an adjacent educational center that focused on animal issues.

Emily, once an anonymous dairy cow, came to be an individual who inspired compassion in the many lives she touched. People from around the world reported that they stopped eating meat simply from learning about her. Their carnistic defenses broke down and were replaced by compassion. Why else would a community of carnists and farmers aid a runaway cow in her flight from slaughter? Why else would the owner of a slaughterhouse donate his cow to an animal sanctuary that doubled as a vegetarian education center?

Emily lived out the rest of her life at the Peace Abbey and died of uterine cancer at the age of ten. Her memorial service attracted international attention, and the testimonials lasted for over an hour. One testimonial in particular captured the essence of Emily's story:

> You catalyzed a new awareness in people by your very presence. One look into your large, luminous brown eyes communicated so much more than words ever could. . . . You gave wordless testimony to the urgent necessity for an all-embracing compassion. . . . There can be no "final re-

spects" to you, Emily, and there can be no closure until the last slaughterhouse has closed its doors, until all beings show compassion to each other, locally and globally. This is a process that will outlive me, too. Your courageous life journey will be an ongoing reminder that I must never give up. You never did.[94]

And Emily's life journey continues to be a reminder. It reminds us to refuse to allow the violent system that is carnism to blind us to the truth, the truth of the needless suffering of billions of animals— and the truth that *we care.*

Emily is immortalized by a life-sized bronze statue in her likeness that stands above her grave at the Peace Abbey. This statue, inscribed with "Emily the Sacred Cow," stands as witness to the billions of animals who are the nameless victims of carnism and to the countless humans who are fighting for their freedom. The statue of the sacred cow embodies the sacred act of bearing witness.

Seeing with the Heart: The Power of Witnessing

When I last visited the Peace Abbey, I stood before each of its monuments. As I gazed up at the towering statue of Gandhi, I saw the world as he had—replete with violence and suffering, but also a place of great beauty and potential. I recalled the 1930 Salt March, and I thought of the dignity of the Indians who gave their lives in the name of nonviolent liberation. I again considered this paradox of the human experience when I looked down at the headstone-like monument inscribed "Innocent Civilians Killed in War." I envisioned the streets of Iraq, the fields of Cambodia, and the jungles of Nicaragua, littered with bodies of all shapes, sizes, colors, and ages. But, too, I remembered the 400,000 people I marched with through the frozen streets of New York City on February 15, 2003, in a peaceful demonstration against the impending invasion of Iraq. Then, as I regarded the statue of Emily, I imagined what it had been like for her, brought into this world to serve as a living machine. I thought of the dark factories, and the terror and helplessness of the countless animals within. But I also thought of the undercover investigators from the Humane Society of the United States, whose videotaping of the brutal mishandling of animals at a slaughterhouse led to public outrage and the largest beef recall in U.S. history. At each monument, I saw the world through the eyes of those it commemorated. I became a witness.

When we bear witness, we are not merely acting as observers; we emotionally connect with the experience of those we are witnessing. We *empathize*. And in so doing, we close the gap in our consciousness, the gap that enables the violence of carnism to endure.

We discussed this gap in our consciousness in chapter 1. It is the missing link in our perception, our failure to connect meat with its animal source. The gap blocks our disgust and our empathy. And it blocks our awareness of the incongruence between our values and our behaviors when it comes to eating meat. Witnessing closes the gap because it connects us with the truth. When we witness, we validate, or make real, the suffering the system works so hard to hide, and we also validate our authentic reaction to it. Witnessing connects us with the truth of carnistic practices, as well as with our inner truth, our empathy. We bear witness to others, and to ourselves.

Just as individual witnessing closes the gap in our consciousness, *collective witnessing* closes the gap in social consciousness. Collective witnessing leads to an informed public and a system in which values and practices are more aligned. Think about it: virtually every atrocity in the history of humankind was enabled by a populace that turned away from a reality that seemed too painful to face, while virtually every revolution for peace and justice has been made possible by a group of people who chose to bear witness and demanded that others bear witness as well. The goal of all justice movements is to activate collective witnessing so that social practices reflect social values. A movement succeeds when it reaches a critical mass of witnesses—that is, enough witnesses to tip the scales of power in favor of the movement. Because mass witnessing is the single greatest threat to carnism, the entire system is organized around preventing this process. Indeed, the sole purpose of carnistic defenses is to block witnessing.

Witnessing can take many forms, including demonstrations, candlelight vigils, banners, lectures, and artistic creations. Witnessing has historically been a creative act: consider the revolutionary music of the 1960s; the AIDS Quilt, which spans a distance of 52.25 miles and bears over 91,000 names; the massive Vietnam Veterans' Memorial wall, which attracts 3 million visitors every year; the largest ever human peace sign, comprised of 6,000 individuals gathered in Ithaca, New York; and Earth Hour 2008, in which 50 million people across seven continents turned off their lights for one hour to show their support for environmental justice.

Witnessing, an act of creation, seems a natural human response to the destruction that it seeks to transform. As renowned psychiatrist Judith Herman tells us, "The ordinary response to atrocities is to banish them from consciousness. . . . Atrocities, however, refuse to be buried. Equally as powerful as the desire to deny atrocities is the conviction that denial does not work."[95] Herman goes on to say that the power of speaking the unspeakable lifts the barriers of denial and repression, releasing tremendous creative energy.

Wired to Care?

Recent research suggests that there may be a biological basis for empathy. In other words, humans (as well as some other animals) may be inherently empathic. Scientists have found that our mirror neurons, neurons in our brain that fire in response to actions, can be activated whether we are performing the actions or simply witnessing them.[96] For example, seeing someone kicking a ball, crying, being harmed, or squirming with an insect crawling up his or her leg activates the same areas of our brain as those that would be activated if the events were happening directly to us. So, to some degree, we know what another feels not simply because we try to put ourselves in his or her shoes, but also because we are literally feeling the same thing.

The implications of these findings are significant. If empathy is hardwired in our brains, an automatic response, then our natural state is one of feeling for others. It may be that when we fail to empathize, we are in fact overriding a natural impulse. Carnistic defenses, then, may actually go against our nature.

From Apathy to Empathy

All violent systems are threatened by mass witnessing because their survival depends on its opposite: mass *dissociation*. Dissociation is the core defense of carnism, the heart of psychic numbing; all other defenses support this central mechanism. Dissociation is psychologically and emotionally disconnecting from the truth of our experience; it is the feeling of not being fully "present" or conscious.

Like other mechanisms, dissociation is at times *adaptive,* or beneficial. For instance, when an individual is being victimized, he or she often automatically dissociates so as not to be overwhelmed by the stress. He or she may describe this sensation as feeling "spaced out" or as an "out-of-body experience." But like other mechanisms, dissociation can be *maladaptive;* it can be used to perpetuate, rather than respond to, violence. In its most extreme form, dissociation can enable a perpetrator to develop a double identity, another "self" that takes over when violating others. Psychiatrist Robert Jay Lifton discusses this phenomenon in his book *The Nazi Doctors,* where he describes medical doctors who worked as killers by day, but were able to return home to their families as seemingly normal husbands and fathers. Most of us, however, don't dissociate to the degree necessary to kill others; we simply dissociate enough to support the killing that is carried out by others. When it comes to eating meat, dissociation prevents us from connecting the dots between what we're doing and how we might actually be feeling. Dissociation essentially renders us powerless to make choices that reflect what we truly feel.

It should come as no surprise that the animals we eat aren't the only ones who pay the price of our dissociation. Dissociation limits our self-awareness and thus presents an obstacle to our personal growth. Virtually all psychological and spiritual traditions consider self-connection, or *integration,* the goal of human development. Integration is the synthesis of different aspects of ourselves into a harmonious whole: body, mind, and spirit; id, ego, and superego; values, beliefs, and behaviors; and so on. Like dissociation, integration is not an all-or-nothing phenomenon. It exists on a continuum. The more integrated we are, the more consistent our character is. For instance, if we're adequately integrated, we aren't fundamentally different people in the workplace than we are at home or with our friends.

Witnessing cultivates integration, as it is an act of connecting. This happens on an individual level, as we connect to our internal experience, and also on a social level, as we connect to the experience of others. This is why witnessing is the Achilles' heel of carnism: it dispels dissociation and leads to a more integrated society. An integrated society cannot consist of people who care about animals and still support widespread animal cruelty.

Witnessing Our Resistance

Despite the transformational power of witnessing, many people resist bearing witness to the reality of carnism. In order to overcome this resistance, we must understand its sources—we must witness our resistance.

The most obvious reason for our resistance is that the system is set up to fortify it. In chapter 5 we discussed how dominant systems shape our thoughts, feelings, and behaviors by laying out invisible "paths of least resistance" for us to follow. These paths dictate the "normal" way to be, which means believing and acting in accordance with the tenets of the system. Dominant systems maintain their dominance by coercing us to conform to the norm. To witness is to deviate from the path of least resistance.

Another reason we resist bearing witness to the truth of carnism is that witnessing hurts. Becoming aware of the intense suffering of billions of animals, and of our own participation in that suffering, can bring up painful emotions: sorrow and grief for the animals; anger at the injustice and deception of the system; despair at the enormity of the problem; fear that trusted authorities and institutions are, in fact, untrustworthy; and guilt for having contributed to the problem. Bearing witness means choosing to suffer. Indeed, empathy is literally "feeling with." Choosing to suffer is particularly difficult in a culture that is addicted to comfort—a culture that teaches that pain should be avoided whenever possible and that ignorance is bliss. We can reduce our resistance to witnessing by valuing authenticity over personal pleasure, and integration over ignorance.

A related reason we resist witnessing the truth of carnism is that we feel powerless to change suffering of such magnitude. It is all too easy to feel discouraged if we believe that "fixing" a problem means that change must be immediate and total. Consider, though, the example of Farm Sanctuary: today it is one of the nation's leading farmed-animal protection organizations, with over 200,000 members and supporters. But it began with just two activists selling vegetarian hot dogs out of their Volkswagen van in 1986. In fact, the very act of witnessing is an act of empowerment; if nothing else, it effects immediate change in *ourselves,* by integrating our values and practices. As vegetarian activist Eddie Lama points out, "I realize that animals will continue to suffer and die—but not because of *me*."[97]

There's a final, perhaps more fundamental, reason we resist witnessing the truth of carnism: if we no longer feel entitled to kill and consume animals, our identity as human beings comes into question. Witnessing compels us to view ourselves as strands in the web of life, rather than as standing at the apex of the so-called food chain. Witnessing challenges our sense of human superiority; it forces us to acknowledge our interconnectedness with the rest of the natural world, an interconnectedness our species has made every effort to deny for thousands of years. And yet witnessing is ultimately liberating. When we recognize that we aren't isolated fragments in a disconnected world, but rather are a part of a vast, living collective, we connect with a power much greater than our individual selves. We no longer support a system that is based on domination and subjugation, a system that follows Hitler's credo that "he who does not possess power loses the right to life."[98] We learn, as author Matthew Scully says, not to measure our lives "in things appropriated, crushed, and killed."[99]

The paradox is that the very reason we resist bearing witness to the truth of carnism is the same reason we desire to witness: because we *care*. This is the great truth that lies buried beneath the elaborate, labyrinthine mechanisms of the system. Because we care, we want to turn away. And because we care, we feel compelled to bear witness. The way to overcome this paradox is to integrate our witnessing: *we must witness the truth of carnism while witnessing ourselves*. We must extend to ourselves the same compassion we allow ourselves to feel for the animals. When we compassionately witness ourselves, we witness our feelings, but without judgment. We recognize ourselves as victims in a system that has led us down the path of least resistance. But we also recognize that we have the power to choose a different path: we have the opportunity to make our choices freely, without the psychological constraints of a covert and coercive system.

Witnessing the Zeitgeist

Despite the extensive reach of carnism, there is reason to believe that the system will destabilize, and the timing is ripe to push for transformation. There are several reasons that challenging carnism is timely: increased awareness of the environmental crisis, a growing concern with animal welfare, the increasing credibility and popularity of vegetarianism, and the unequaled availability of information on both carnism and vegetarianism.

Widescale meat production is a leading cause of environmental destruction.[100] Methane gasses emitted from thousands of pounds of manure deplete the ozone layer. Toxic runoff from tons of chemicals used on the animals—synthetic hormones, antibiotics, pesticides, and fungicides—pollute the air and waterways. Thousands of acres of woodlands are clear-cut to allow for the planting of feed crops, leading to topsoil erosion and deforestation. More fresh water is usurped from reservoirs than can be replenished. And chemical fertilizers seep into rivers and streams, enabling the proliferation of microorganisms that destroy aquatic life. Leading scientists agree that the system of mass meat production cannot continue without causing a breakdown of the ecosystem. Environmental protection has become an increasingly important concern of Americans, as can be seen through the proliferation of "green" products, publications, and policies. As Americans become more concerned about ecological sustainability, they invariably become more concerned about carnistic practices.

Perhaps not coincidentally, Americans have also become more concerned with animal welfare. This is demonstrated by the countless animal protection organizations that have sprung up across the country. And despite the fact that animal welfare advocacy has typically applied to only those species we consider pets, it is expanding to include other animals as well. For instance, the largest animal protection organization in the country, the Humane Society of the United States, now boasts an entire division dedicated to the protection of farmed animals. And People for the Ethical Treatment of Animals (PETA), a more radical and openly anticarnist organization, has become a household name.

Moreover, vegetarianism, once considered an extreme ideology and a diet of questionable nutritional soundness, is making its way into the mainstream. While vegetarians still make up a minority of the population, and many health professionals still cling to carnistic myths, those who eschew meat are less often marginalized and pathologized than they would have been just a decade ago. The face of vegetarianism is no longer the flower child of the 1960s; celebrities from Sir Paul McCartney to Bill Pearl, bodybuilder and five-time Mr. Universe, are ambassadors for a diverse, growing movement. And more and more studies have compelled the medical community to admit that not only can a plant-based diet be as healthful as a meat-based one, but there's a good chance it's even healthier. Indeed, the proliferation of vegetarian publications, food products, and organizations suggests that the movement is increasing in size and strength. Anyone who doubts this need only open the dictionary to find that it now includes the term "vegan"—a person who eschews all animal products.

A final reason that the timing is ripe to challenge carnism is that the primary defense of the system, invisibility, has been weakening. It is becoming increasingly difficult for carnistic industries to hide their secrets from the public; the animal agribusinesses that depend on controlling information to sustain the myths of meat are now challenged by a ubiquitous, unregulated information source: the Internet. Carnism is like the Wizard of Oz: once the curtain is pulled back from the system, its power virtually disappears.

> **Threats Are REAL**
> **Threats Are NOW**
> **Potential Impact Is Enormous**
>
> —Slide at the end of a PowerPoint presentation entitled *Animal Welfare and Activism: What You Need to Know,* from the 2008 Food Marketing Institute/American Meat Institute Meat Conference

Witnessing in Action: What You Can Do

As I mentioned earlier, witnessing the extensive suffering inherent in carnism can cause one to feel helpless and frustrated. But there *are* things you can do that will directly impact your own life and the lives of farmed animals, and to that end I've provided a list of resources at the back of this book.

There are three important steps you can take to get started: eliminate or reduce your consumption of animal products, support an advocacy organization, and continue to inform yourself and others. While eliminating your consumption of animal products is ideal, just reducing the amount of them in your diet can have a significant impact on the animals and on yourself; for instance, a person who eats meat once or twice a month consumes far fewer animals than someone who eats meat daily. Clearly, this helps the animals. But you, too, benefit, as you feel more integrated in your values and practices.

And you don't need to work toward change on your own. Millions of people around the world are actively working to abolish carnism, and it's easier than ever to join up with them. If a vegetarian group or animal advocacy organization doesn't exist in your region, you can connect with one through the Internet. Getting involved with an organization gives you options for contributing to the cause. You can donate money, help with advocacy efforts, or do any number of things to help reduce animal suffering.

Perhaps most importantly, you can and should continue to learn and teach others. It's all too easy to forget, to fall back into the cocoon of psychic numbing. Remember: your carnistic schema will pull you back into the carnistic mentality; your awareness of meat production will diminish if you don't actively work to keep yourself informed and try to deepen your understanding of the issue.* Make witnessing your credo.

---

*Staying informed does *not* mean continually exposing yourself to graphic imagery. Once you're aware of the suffering of farmed animals, you don't need to expose yourself to potentially traumatizing information.

Beyond Carnism

The mechanisms that enable widescale meat consumption are not unique to carnism. As I have pointed out, carnism is just one of numerous entrenched, or dominant, ideologies. And any dominant ideology that requires the participation of individuals who, if they were more fully informed, might choose to withhold their support utilizes the same mechanisms as carnism. Thus, understanding carnism can help us think more critically about all systems in which we participate. Consider the arguments and psychology that have enabled widespread hatred and discrimination toward homosexuals, the deeply entrenched system of apartheid, and the genocide in Darfur. In each of these instances, the violence has been denied, justified, and distorted to garner mass support.

The same holds true for witnessing: because destructive ideologies share similar structural features, witnessing carnism can give us a framework for witnessing other systems. Indeed, the ability to witness extends beyond carnism because witnessing isn't merely something one *does;* it is how one *is.* Witnessing isn't an isolated practice, but a way of relating to oneself and the world. It is a way of life that informs our interactions with ourselves and others. And there is no limit to our capacity for witnessing.* In fact, because witnessing is empowering, the more we witness, the greater our ability to witness. Like compassion, our capacity for witnessing grows with practice.

---

*Though witnessing may at times be painful, it should never make you feel emotionally unsafe. Witnessing means staying mentally and emotionally open to the experience of oneself and others; it does not mean forcing yourself to take in deeply distressing information. Many animal advocates become traumatized from overexposing themselves to the horrors of meat production—this kind of witnessing is unnecessary and is ultimately counterproductive.

The Courage to Witness

Bearing witness takes courage. It takes courage to open our hearts to the suffering of others and to acknowledge that, for better or worse, we are part of the system in which that suffering takes place. Indeed, as James O'Dea, former director of Amnesty International, explains:

> The witness stands together, inside, with those who are hurt and with those who are violated; the witness has an extraordinary capacity to stand in the fires of hatred and violence without increasing those elements. In fact, the deepest form of witnessing is a form of compassion for all suffering beings. . . . In reality, we are never outside observers. We are inside the wound together. It is just that some feel and some are numb. We are inside the very thing that needs to be transformed.[101]

Bearing witness takes the courage to refuse to follow the path of least resistance. Like Emily the cow, we have been herded into a lineup, taught to follow a course that's been laid out for us. But like Emily, we can choose to break from the line and shift the trajectory of our lives. Whether or not you were previously aware of the truth of carnism, that you have chosen to read this book is testament to your courage to take the road less traveled. The information in this book is provocative, controversial, and at times deeply disturbing, and it takes courage to witness it.

Bearing witness takes the courage to realize the potential of the human spirit. Witnessing requires us to call forth the highest qualities of our species, qualities such as conviction, integrity, empathy, and compassion. It is easier by far to retain the attributes of carnistic culture: apathy, complacency, self-interest, and "blissful" ignorance. I wrote this book—itself an act of witnessing—because I believe that, as humans, we have a fundamental desire to strive to become our best selves. I believe that each and every one of us has the capacity to act as powerful witnesses in a world very much in need. I have had the opportunity to interact with thousands of individuals through my work as a teacher, author, and speaker, and through my personal life. I have witnessed, again and again, the courage and compassion of the so-called average American: previously apathetic students who become impassioned activists; lifelong carnists who weep openly when exposed to images of animal cruelty, never again to eat meat; butchers who suddenly connect meat to its living source and become unable to continue killing animals; and a community of carnists who aid a runaway cow in her flight from slaughter.

Ultimately, bearing witness requires the courage to take sides. In the face of mass violence, we will inevitably fall into a role: victim or perpetrator. Judith Herman argues that all bystanders are forced to take a side, by their action or inaction, and that there is no such thing as moral neutrality. Indeed, as Nobel Peace Prize Laureate and Holocaust survivor Elie Wiesel points out, "Neutrality helps the oppressor, never the victim. Silence encourages the tormentor, never the tormented."[102] Witnessing enables us to choose our role rather than having one assigned to us. And although those of us who choose to stand with the victim may suffer, as Herman says, "There can be no greater honor."[103]

RESOURCES

I. Transitioning to a Meat-Free Diet

The Ultimate Vegan Guide: Compassionate Living without Sacrifice by Erik Marcus

This short, easily readable book tells readers everything they need to know in order to adopt a healthful, meat-free lifestyle. Topics covered include reasons to stop eating meat, cooking, nutrition, food shopping, dining out, and much more.

Physicians Committee for Responsible Medicine (PCRM)

www.pcrm.org

This website offers vegetarian starter kits, tips for reducing your meat consumption, and a tremendous amount of great health and nutrition information.

Vegetarian Resource Group (VRG)

www.vrg.org

Here you can find answers to FAQs about vegetarian living and nutrition, information on animal ingredients in foods, sample menus, and archived articles on a number of issues pertaining to vegetarianism.

www.NewVeg.av.org

This site is a gold mine of information and it includes tips for transitioning to a meat-free diet, information on gradual versus abrupt dietary changes, how to manage initial cravings, concerns about maintaining a meat-free diet, understanding new feelings about meat and vegetarianism, and much more.

Vegetarian Times Vegetarian Beginner's Guide

This is a great introduction to the vegetarian lifestyle, by the editors of *Vegetarian Times* magazine. It answers questions about vitamin supplements and different types of vegetarianism, and offers ideas for your pantry, recipes, and menus, while debunking misconceptions about vegetarianism. This is a paperback book, available on Amazon.

People for the Ethical Treatment of Animals (PETA)

www.peta.org
www.goveg.com
This is a huge website, full of information on a variety of issues concerning animals. The site offers a vegetarian starter kit, a vegetarian cooking blog, and a host of other resources.

VegFamily

www.vegfamily.com
This excellent online magazine has a plethora of information on vegetarian living for the whole family. There are tips for expectant mothers, raising vegetarian babies and children, and preparing healthy family meals. The site also hosts a discussion forum and offers a wide variety of resources for vegetarians.

Vegetarianteen.com

This site helps vegetarian teens connect with each other and provides a wealth of information of specific interest to young people. There are books and reviews, tips on animal-free clothing, and information for parents who are concerned about their child's choice to stop eating meat.

Dr. John McDougall
www.drmcdougall.com
Dr. McDougall has many articles, books, and DVDs available on healthy vegetarian eating.

II. Vegetarian Substitutes for Animal Products

Today it's possible to find a vegetarian substitute for virtually any animal product. Because every product has a different taste and texture, it's best to try a number of them to see which you prefer. Some are so realistic that even the staunchest of carnists can't tell the difference; others are not intended to seem meatlike. And as with any type of food, these products fall into different price ranges, some being much more affordable than others.

Some of the more "realistic" tasting brands include Boca, Tofurkey, Lightlife, Yves, Tofutti, Field Roast, Silk, So Decadent, Morningstar Farms, Earth Balance, and Vegenaise. On its website (*www.vrg.org*), the Vegetarian Resource Group has a link to a long list of meat, dairy, and egg substitutes. Also, at *www.veganwolf.com,* you can find information about how to convert meat-based recipes to plant-based ones, lists and reviews of substitute foods, and tips on cooking without animal products. A page of the PETA website, *www.peta.org / accidentallyvegan,* lists many commonly consumed items that are made without animal products, from Fritos to Pillsbury pizza dough. And at *www.Vegan-Essentials.com* you can find animal-free products for purchase, from marshmallows to shoes.

Following are some vegetarian substitutes to try:

Animal-Based	Vegetarian
Butter	Earth Balance, Smart Balance
Baking mixes (pancake, cookie, cake)	Cherrybrook Kitchen mixes
Cream cheese	Tofutti or Soy Kaas Cream Cheese
Mayonnaise	Vegenaise or Nayonaise
Eggs (for cooking)	Ener-G Egg Replacer
Yogurt	Soy Yogurt (Trader Joe's, So Delicious, Stonyfield Farm O'Soy, Silk)
Half-and-half	Silk Creamer
Milk	Silk Soy Milk
Whipped cream	Soy Whip
Milk chocolate	Dark chocolate
Hamburger	Boca Burger, Morningstar Farms Griller's Prime
Hot dog	Yves Hot Dogs
Sausage	Field Roast, Tofurkey, Gimme Lean, Morningstar Farms sausages
Chicken nuggets	Boca Chick'n Nuggets (or Patties)
Deli-meat slices	Tofurkey, Lightlife Smart Deli slices
Beef strips/sirloin tips	Morningstar Farms Meal Starters (also comes in chicken strips)
Barbecued ribs	Morningstar Farms Hickory BBQ Riblets

III. Tips for Grocery Shopping and Dining Out

The **Vegetarian Resource Group** offers solutions to common problems with shopping, eating out, and traveling for vegetarians. On its website, it lists vegetarian-friendly chain restaurants, online restaurant guides, and tips for reading food labels when you're avoiding animal products.

The grocery-store chain **Trader Joe's,** at *www.traderjoes.com,* offers printable lists of all vegetarian products it sells. There are copies of this list in the stores as well.

At *www.vegan.com* you can find a list of all ingredients that come from animals or animal by-products, such as whey and tallow.

Most major grocery store chains now carry a number of vegetarian food substitutes, and some products are available for purchase online.

When eating out, it's helpful to know what foods always or often have animal products in them. For example, risotto is virtually always made with cheese, and rice may be cooked in chicken stock. It's always a good idea to call ahead to a restaurant to ask whether they offer vegetarian selections, and, if not, whether the chef would make something up for you. In many restaurants, it isn't a problem to request a vegetarian meal that's made to order.

IV. Organizations Promoting Vegetarianism and Farm-Animal Welfare

There are a wide variety of organizations promoting vegetarianism and farmed animal welfare. Below is a short list of somewhat diverse groups.

Farm Sanctuary

www.farmsanctuary.org

Farm Sanctuary is a farmed animal rescue organization and sanctuary. It provides information on campaigns for farmed animals and also on vegetarianism, education, and advocacy.

The Humane Farming Association

www.hfa.org

This site has information on CAFOs, legislation for farmed animal welfare, boycotts, and opportunities to help improve the lives of farmed animals.

FARM (Farm Animal Rights Movement)

www.farmusa.org

FARM has information on campaigns for farmed animal welfare, vegetarianism, and opportunities for people who want to get involved in the movement.

Jewish Veg

www.jewishveg.com

This site provides information on Judaism and vegetarianism, including information about kosher eating.

The Christian Vegetarian Association

www.christianveg.com

This is a site where Christian vegetarians can meet and find information connecting Christianity and vegetarianism.

International Vegetarian Union

www.ivu.org

This site has information on vegetarianism around the world, including information for vegetarian travelers.

North American Vegetarian Society (NAVS)

www.navs-online.org

NAVS offers outreach material and information on vegetarian events, vegetarian living, and veganic gardening and farming, as well as much more.

Humane Society of the United States (HSUS)

www.hsus.org

The HSUS now has a farmed animal division, which offers a wealth of information on the lives of farmed animals as well as on campaigns and legislation. It also offers a number of vegetarian recipes.

V. Recommended Reading and Viewing

There are countless books and DVDs on vegetarian philosophy, cooking, and health. Below are a few you may want to start with (full citations are in the bibliography).

Living Among Meat Eaters by Carol J. Adams
An excellent book for helping new and seasoned vegetarians cope in a carnistic world. Includes tips for talking to carnists, eating in mixed groups, and finding personal empowerment as a vegetarian.

How to Eat Like a Vegetarian Even If You Never Want To Be One: More Than 250 Shortcuts, Strategies, and Simple Solutions by Patti Breitman and Carol J. Adams
A great guide for beginning vegetarians, with tips on simple ways to make meat-free meals, lists, and charts on nutrition and ingredients, and a host of practical resources for healthful eating.

Thanking the Monkey by Karen Dawn
A thorough, highly praised book on animal welfare issues, including those involving farm animals.

Vegan: The New Ethics of Eating by Erik Marcus
A staple on veganism. Short but full of valuable information.

The Food Revolution by John Robbins
A comprehensive guide to healthy, vegetarian living.

Dominion by Matthew Scully
A "conservative case" for animal rights. Scully argues why political conservatives must concern themselves with the welfare of animals.

Animal Liberation by Peter Singer

A classic and staple for anyone interested in animal welfare.

Dr. Michael Greger's nutrition and health DVDs

The most engaging, entertaining, and informative selection of DVDs on the dangers of consuming animal products and the benefits of vegetarianism. Available at *www.drgreger.org*.

Tribe of Heart DVDs

Deeply moving documentaries about the lives of animals exploited by humans. Available at *www.tribeofheart.org*.

Food, Inc.

A powerful documentary by filmmaker Robert Kenner on the animal agribusiness industry. Features Eric Schlosser and Michael Pollan.

NOTES

1 Lotte Holm and M. Mohl, "The Role of Meat in Everyday Food Culture: An Analysis of an Interview Study in Copenhagen," *Appetite* 34 (2000): 277–283.

2 Nick Fiddes, *Meat: A Natural Symbol* (New York: Rutledge, 1991); Peter Farb and George Armelagos, *Consuming Passions: The Anthropology of Eating* (Boston: Houghton Mifflin, 1980); Frederick J. Simoons, *Eat Not This Flesh: Food Avoidances in the Old World* (Madison: University of Wisconsin Press, 1961); "Food Taboos: It's All a Matter of Taste," *National Geographic News, http://news.nationalgeographic.com/news/2004/04/0419_040419_TVfoodtaboo.html*; Fessler, Daniel, M. T. Navarrette, and Carlos David Navarrette. "Meat Is Good to Taboo: Dietary Proscriptions as a Product of the Interaction of Psychological Mechanisms and Social Processes," *Journal of Cognition and Culture* 3.1 (2003): 1–40, *http://www.sscnet.ucla.edu/anthro/faculty/fessler/pubs/MeatIsGoodToTaboo.pdf* (accessed 26 Mar. 2009).

3 Farb and Armelagos; Simoons; Daniel Kelly, "The Role of Psychology in the Study of Culture," *Purdue University,* available at *http://web.ics.purdue.edu/~drkelly/KellyMacheryMallon MasonStichCommentonMesoudietal.htm* (accessed 26 Mar. 2009).

4 Cited in Dave Grossman, *On Killing: The Psychological Cost of Learning to Kill in War and Society.* (New York: Back Bay Books, 1996), 12.

5 Grossman; Martha Stout, *The Sociopath Next Door.* (New York: Broadway Books, 2005).

6 Grossman, 15.

7   See Humane Society of the United States statistics on factory
     farming for statistics on meat consumption and animal slaugh-
     ter, available at *http://www.hsus.org/farm*.

8   U.S. Department of Agriculture, Grain Inspection, Packers,
     and Stockyards Administration (GIPSA), 30 Mar. 2009, *http://
     www.gipsa.usda.gov/GIPSA/webapp?area=newsroom&subject=
     landing&topic=cc-budget-03*. Statement of David R. Shipman,
     acting administrator of the Grain Inspection, Packers, and
     Stockyards Administration, before the Subcommittee on Agri-
     culture, Rural Development, and Related Agencies, in refer-
     ence to the FY 2003 budget proposal.

9   Daniel Zwerdling, "A View to a Kill," *Gourmet* (June 2007),
     available at *http://www.gourmet.com/magazine/2000s/2007/06/
     aviewtoakill* (accessed 26 Mar. 2009). Also see Kim Severson,
     "Upton Sinclair, Now Playing on YouTube," *The New York Times*,
     12 Mar. 2008, available at *http://www.nytimes.com/2008/
     03/12/dining/12animal.html?pagewanted=2&_r=1* (accessed 26
     Mar. 2009).

10   Eric Schlosser, "Fast Food Nation: Meat and Potatoes," *Rolling
     Stone*, 3 Sep. 1998, available at *http://www.ericsecho.org/
     investigation2.htm* (accessed 13 Mar. 2009).

11   Study cited by the Humane Society of the United States, available
     at *http://www.hsus.org/farm/resources/animals/pigs/pigs.html*.

12   For information on PSS, see Tammy McCormick Donaldson, "Is
     Boredom Driving Pigs Crazy?" The University of Idaho College
     of Natural Resources, available at *http://www.cnr.uidaho.edu/
     range556/Appl_BEHAVE/projects/pigs_ster.html* (accessed 26 Mar.
     2009), and Wayne Du, "Porcine Stress Syndrome Gene and Pork
     Production," Ontario Ministry of Agriculture Food and Rural Af-
     fairs, June 2004, available at *http://www.omafra.gov.on.ca/english/
     livestock/swine/facts/04-053.htm* (accessed 27 Mar. 2009). For
     information on the genetic basis of PTSD, see Aimee Midei,
     "Identification of the First Gene in Posttraumatic Stress Disorder,"
     Bio-medicine.org, 22 Sep. 2002, *http://news.bio-medicine.org/*

biology-news-2/Identification-of-the-first-gene-in-posttraumatic-stress-disorder-6692-1/ ... (accessed 27 Mar. 2009).

13 Wayne Du, Ontario Ministry of Agriculture Food and Rural Affairs, June 2004, available at *http://www.omafra.gov.on.ca/english/livestock/swine/facts/04-053.htm* (accessed 27 Mar. 2009).

14 Joe Vansickle, "Preparing Pigs for Transport," *The National Hog Farmer,* 15 Sep. 2008, available at *http://nationalhogfarmer.com/behavior-welfare/0915-preparing-pigs-transport/* (accessed 26 Mar. 2009).

15 Gail Eisnitz, *Slaughterhouse:The Shocking Story of Greed, Neglect, and Inhumane Treatment Inside the U.S. Meat Industry* (Amherst, NY: Prometheus Books, 1997), 102–104.

16 Schlosser, "Fast Food Nation: Meat and Potatoes."

17 Eisnitz, 68.

18 Ibid., 84.

19 Eisnitz, 93.

20 David Irvin, "Control Debate, Growers Advised," *Arkansas-Democrat Gazette,* Northwest Arkansas edition, 22 Sep. 2007, available at *http://www.nwanews.com/adg/Business/202171/* (accessed 26 Mar. 2009).

21 Cited in Joan Dunayer, *Animal Equality: Language and Liberation,* (Derwood, MD: Ryce Publishing, 2001), 138.

22 Ibid., 137.

23 Ibid.

24 Cited in Fiddes, 96.

25 Michael Pollan, *The Omnivore's Dilemma:A Natural History of Four Meals* (New York: Penguin, 2006), 72.

26 Ibid., 69.

27 See Clyde Lane, Jr., et al., "Castration of Beef Calves," *TheBeefSite.com: TheWebsite for the Global Beef Industry,* January 2007, *http://www.thebeefsite.com/articles/930/castration-of-beef-calves.*

28 Michael Pollan, "Power Steer," *The New York Times,* sec. 6, 31 Mar. 2002; "Pollution from Giant Livestock Farms Threatens Public Health," National Resources Defense Council, 15 July 2005, *http://www.nrdc.org/water/pollution/nspills.asp* (accessed 26 Mar. 2009).

29 Eisnitz, 46.

30 Ibid., 43–44.

31 Schlosser, "Fast Food Nation: Meat and Potatoes."

32 Joby Warrick, "They Die Piece by Piece," *The Washington Post,* 10 Apr. 2001, available at *http://www.hfa.org/hot_topic/wash_post.pdf* (accessed 26 Mar. 2009).

33 See Sandra Blakeslee, "Minds of Their Own: Birds Gain Respect," *The New York Times,* 1 Feb. 2005, available at *http://www.nytimes.com/2005/02/01/science/01bird.html* (accessed 31 Mar. 2009).

34 Josh Balk, "COK Investigation Exposes Chicken Industry Cruelty; Undercover Footage of Perdue Slaughter Plant Reveals Routine Abuse," Compassion Over Killing, *http://www.cok.net/camp/inv/perdue/notes.php.*

35 For information on pain studies discussed in this section, see K. J. S. Anand, D. Phil, and P. R. Hickey, "Pain and Its Effects in the Human Neonate and Fetus," *CIRP.org:* The Circumcision Reference Library, 5 Sep. 2006, available at *http://www.cirp.org/library/pain/anand/* (accessed 27 Mar. 2009); K. J. S. Anand, D. Phil, and P. R. Hickey. "Pain and Its Effects in the Human Neonate and Fetus." *New England Journal of Medicine* 317. 21 (Nov. 1987): 1321–1329. *http://www.cirp.org/library/pain/anand/* (accessed 27 Mar. 2009).

Liz Austin, "Whole Foods Bans Sale of Live Lobsters," *CBSnews.com,* 16 June 2006, *http://www.cbsnews.com/stories/2006/06/16/ap/business/mainD8I99PROO.shtml* (accessed 27 Mar. 2009); David B. Chamberlain, "Babies Remember Pain," *CIRP.org:* The Circumcision Reference Library, 15 Dec. 2006. *http://www.cirp.org/library/psych/chamberlain/* (accessed 27

Mar. 2009); David B. Chamberlain. "Babies Remember Pain," *Journal of Prenatal and Perinatal Psychology and Health* 3. 4 (1989): 297–310, *http://www.cirp.org/library/psych/chamberlain* (accessed 27 Mar. 2009).

J. P. Chambers, et al., "Self-Selection of the Analgesic Drug Carprofen by Lame Broiler Chickens," *The Veterinary Record* 146.11 (2000): 307–311. See also Mary T. Phillips, "Savages, Drunks, and Lab Animals: The Researcher's Perception of Pain," *Society and Animals* 1.1 (1993): 61–81.

36 Jia-rui Chong, "Wood-Chipped Chickens Fuel Outrage," *Los Angeles Times,* 22 Nov. 2003, available at *http://articles.latimes.com/2003/nov/22/local/me-chipper22* (accessed 26 Mar. 2009).

37 American Veterinary Medical Association, "Welfare Implications of the Veal Calf Husbandry," 13 Oct. 2008, available at *http://www.avma.org/issues/animal_welfare/veal_calf_husbandry_bgnd.asp* (accessed 27 Mar. 2009).

38 Eisnitz, 43.

39 For information in this section on the cognitive abilities of sea animals, see the Humane Society of the United States website, available at *http://www.hsus.org/farm/resources/animals/*. Also see Culum Brown, Kevin Laland, and Jens Krause, eds., Fish Cognition and Behavior (Oxford, UK: Blackwell Publishing, 2006), for an in-depth discussion of the cognitive abilities of fish; and Jeffrey Masson, *The Face on Your Plate: The Truth About Food* (New York: W.W. Norton, 2009).

40 For information in this section on the sentience of sea animals, see "Fish May Actually Feel Pain and React to It Much Like Humans Do," *Science Daily,* 1 May 2009, *http://www.sciencedaily.com/releases/2009/04/090430161242.htm* (accessed 4 June 2009). This article gives a detailed description of the study on goldfish's response to increased temperatures. Also see Alex Kirby, "Fish Do Feel Pain, Scientists Say," BBC News Online, *http://news.bbc.co.uk/2/hi/science/nature/2983045.stm* (accessed 4 June 2009). This article discusses the first conclusive

evidence of pain receptors in fish, and describes the study where fish's lips were injected with an acidic substance. The original article on fish lip injection is from L.U. Sneddon, V. A. Braithwaite, and M. J. Gentle, "Do Fishes Have Nociceptors? Evidence for the Evolution of a Vertebrate Sensory System," *Proceedings of the Royal Society of London,* B 270. 1520 (7 June 2003): 1115–1121.

41 For information on commercial and farm fishing, see Ken Jacobsen and Linda Riebel, *Eating to Save the Earth: Food Choices for a Healthy Planet* (Berkley, CA: Celestial Arts, 2002). Also see Marcus, *Meat Market;* the Humane Society of the United States at *http://www.hsus.org/farm/resources/animals/*; and Masson.

42 For information on legislation regarding nonambulatory live-stock, see "Judge Rules Recumbent Pigs May Be Processed," *Thepigsite.com,* 3 Feb. 2009, *http://www.thepigsite.com/swinenews/20475/judge-rules-recumbent-pigs-may-be-processed;* The Humane Society of the United States, Factory Farming Campaign, *http://www.hsus.org/farm.*

43 Damien McElroy, "Korean Outrage as West Tries to Use World Cup to Ban Dog Eating," *Telegraph,* 6 Jan. 2002, available at *http://www.telegraph.co.uk/news/worldnews/europe/france/1380569/Korean-outrage-as-West-tries-to-use-World-Cup-to-ban-dog-eating.html* (accessed 26 Mar. 2009).

44 LJ, "Stop the Dog Meat Industry," ASPCA Online Community, 18 Feb. 2009, *http://aspcacommunity.ning.com/forum/topics/stop-the-dog-meat-industry* (accessed 26 Mar. 2009).

45 Schlosser, "Fast Food Nation: Meat and Potatoes."

46 See Dan Morgan, Gilbert M. Gaul, and Sarah Cohen, "Harvesting Cash: A Year-Long Investigation into Farm Subsidies," *The Washington Post,* 2006, available at *http://www.washingtonpost.com/wp-srv/nation/interactives/farmaid/* (accessed 25 Mar. 2009). Also see "EWG Farm Bill 2007 Policy Analysis Database," Environmental Working Group, *http://farm.ewg.org/sites/farmbill2007/* (accessed 25 Mar. 2009).

47   For information on working conditions in the meatpacking in-
     dustry, see Human Rights Watch, "Blood, Sweat and Fear," *HRW.
     org,* 24 Jan. 2005, *http://www.hrw.org/en/node/11869/section/5*
     (accessed 27 Mar. 2009); Lance Compa and Jamie Fellner,
     "Meatpacking's Human Toll," *The Washington Post,* 3 Aug. 2005,
     available at *http://www.washingtonpost.com/wp-dyn/content/
     article/2005/08/02/AR2005080201936.html* (accessed 27 Mar.
     2009); Megan Feldman, "Swift Meat Packing Plant and Illegal
     Immigrants," *The Houston Press,* 4 Apr. 2007, available at *http://
     www.houstonpress.com/2007-04-05/news/swift-meatpacking-plant-
     and-illegal-immigrants/* (accessed 27 Mar. 2009); Jeremy Rifkin,
     Beyond Beef; Eric Schlosser, *Fast Food Nation: The Dark Side of the
     All-American Meal* (New York: Houghton Mifflin, 2001).

48   For information on the effects of CAFOs on human health, see
     Mark Bittman, "Rethinking the Meat-Guzzler," *The New York
     Times,* 27 Jan. 2008, available at *http://www.nytimes.com/
     2008/01/27/weekinreview/27bittman.html?_r=2* (accessed 26
     Mar. 2009); Jennifer Lee, "Neighbors of Vast Hog Farms Say
     Foul Air Endangers Their Health," *The New York Times,* 11 May
     2003, available online at *http://www.nytimes.com/2003/05/11/
     us/neighbors-of-vast-hog-farms-say-foul-air-endangers-their-health.
     html* (accessed 26 Mar. 2009); Pollan, "Power Steer"; National
     Resources Defense Council, "Pollution from Giant Livestock
     Farms Threatens Public Health," 15 July 2005, *http://
     www.nrdc.org/water/pollution/nspills.asp* (accessed 26 Mar.,
     2009); and Johns Hopkins Bloomberg School of Public Health,
     "Public Health Association Calls for Moratorium on Factory
     Farms; Cites Health Issues, Pollution," 9 Jan. 2004, *http://
     www.jhsph.edu/publichealthnews/press_releases/PR_2004/farm_
     moratorium.html* (accessed 26 Mar. 2009).

49   See Michael Greger, *Bird Flu: A Virus of Our Own Hatching* (New
     York: Lantern Books, 2006); Rifkin; and Union of Concerned
     Scientists, "They Eat What? The Reality of Feed at Animal

Factories," *UCSUSA.org,* 8 Aug. 2006, *http://www.ucsusa.org/food_and_agriculture/science_and_impacts/impacts_industrial_agriculture/they-eat-what-the-reality-of.html* (accessed 27 Mar. 2009).

50 Cited in Justin Ewers, "Don't Read This Over Dinner," *U.S. News and World Report,* 7 Aug. 2005, available at *http://www.usnews.com/usnews/culture/articles/050815/15meat.htm* (accessed 31 Mar. 2009).

51 WGBH Educational Foundation, "What Is HAACP," available at *http://www.pbs.org/wgbh/pages/frontline/shows/meat/evaluating/haccp.html* (accessed 27 Mar. 2009). Also see Rifkin.

52 Greger. S. Pao, M., M.R. Ettinger, MF Khalid, AO Reid, and BL Nerrie, "Microbial quality of raw aquacultured fish fillets procured from Internet and local retail markets," *Journal of Food Protection,* Aug. 2008 71. 8:1844–1849.

53 Greger.

54 Rifkin, 140.

55 Stephen J. Hedges and Washington Bureau, "E. Coli Loophole Cited in Recalls Tainted Meat Can Be Sold if Cooked," *Chicago Tribune,* 11 Nov. 2007, available at *http://archives.chicagotribune.com/2007/nov/11/food/chi-meat_bdnov11* (accessed 27 Mar. 2009).

56 Human Rights Watch.

57 See Karen Gaudette, "USDA Expands Ground-Beef Recall," *The Seattle Times,* 4 July 2008, available at *http://seattletimes.nwsource.com/html/nationworld/2008033109_beefrecall04.html* (accessed 27 Mar. 2009); "Nebraska Beef Recalls 1.2 Million Pounds of Beef," *MSNBC.com,* 10 Aug. 2008, *http://www.msnbc.msn.com/id/26101733/* (accessed 27 Mar. 2009); and U.S. Department of Agriculture, "Nebraska Firm Recalls Beef Products Due to Possible E. coli O157:H7 Contamination," 30 June 2008, available at *http://www.fsis.usda.gov/News_&_Events/Recall_022_2008_?Release/index.asp* (accessed 27 Mar. 2009).

58 Stephen J. Hedges and Washington Bureau, "Topps Meat Recall Raises Questions About Inspections Workload," *Chicago*

Tribune, 14 Oct. 2007, available at *http://archives.chicagotribune
.com/2007/oct/14/food/chi-meat_5s_hedgesoct14* (accessed 27
Mar. 2009).

59 Schlosser, "Fast Food Nation: Meat and Potatoes."

60 Eric Schlosser, "The Chain Never Stops," *Mother Jones,* July/Aug.
2001, available at *http://www.motherjones.com/news/
feature/2001/07/meatpacking.html* (accessed 27 Mar. 2009).

61 Ibid.

62 Human Rights Watch.

63 Eisnitz, 87.

64 Ibid.

65 Ibid.

66 Ibid., 94.

67 Frederic J. Frommer, "Video Shows Workers Abusing Pigs,"
The Guardian Unlimited, 17 Sep. 2008, available at *http://
www.guardian.co.uk/uslatest/story/0,,-7805670,00.html*
(accessed 31 Mar. 2009).

68 See Fiddes and Simoons.

69 For information on the environmental effects of the meatpacking
industry, see Jacobsen and Riebel; Food and Agriculture Organization of the United Nations, "Livestock's Long Shadow: Environmental Issues and Options," 2006, available at *http://www.fao.org/
docrep/010/a0701e/a0701e00.HTM* (accessed 27 Mar. 2009);
and Union of Concerned Scientists, *www.ucsusa.org.*

70 Johns Hopkins Bloomberg School of Public Health.

71 Center for Science in the Public Interest, *http://www.cspinet.
org/*; Jacobsen and Riebel, *Eating to Save the Earth*; and Food and
Agriculture Organization of the United Nations, "Livestock's
Long Shadow: Environmental Issues and Options."

72 See William Heffernan and Mary Hendrickson, "Concentration
of Agricultural Markets," *National Farmer's Union,* Apr. 2007,
http://www.nfu.org/wp-content/2007-heffernanreport.pdf (accessed 25 Mar. 2009).

73 Philip Mattera, "USDA Inc.: How Agribusiness Has Hijacked
Regulatory Policy at the U.S. Department of Agriculture,"

Corporate research project of Good Jobs First, 23 July 2004, *http://www.agribusinessaccountability.org/pdfs/289_USDA%20 Inc..pdf* (accessed 25 Mar. 2009).

74 Ibid.

75 Marion Nestle, *Food Politics: How the Food Industry Influences Nutrition and Health* (Berkeley: University of California Press, 2007) and Center for Responsive Politics, "Money in Politics—See Who's Giving and Who's Getting," available at *http://www.opensecrets.org/index.php* (accessed 25 Mar. 2009).

76 Doug Gurian-Sherman, "CAFOs Uncovered: The Untold Costs of Confined Animal Feeding Operations," Union of Concerned Scientists, Apr. 2008, *http://www.ucsusa.org/assets/documents/food_and_agriculture/cafos-uncovered-executive-summary.pdf* (accessed 31 Mar. 2009).

77 See Joe Ruff, "ConAgra Chief's Compensation Tops $10 Million," *Omaha World Herald,* 17 Aug. 2007, available at *http://www.omaha.com/index.php?u_page=1208&u_sid=10109885* (accessed 31 Mar. 2009).

78 See Centers for Disease Control, "Multistate Outbreak of *Escherichia coli* O157:H7 Infections Associated with Eating Ground Beef—United States, June–July 2002," 26 July 2002, available at *http://www.cdc.gov/mmwr/preview/mmwrhtml/mm5129a1.htm* (accessed 31 Mar. 2009); see also "About E. Coli," *http://www.about-ecoli.com/ecoli_outbreaks/view/conagra-e-coli-outbreak*.

79 R. L. Phillips, "Coronary Heart Disease Mortality Among Seventh Day Adventists with Differing Dietary Habits: A Preliminary Report," *Cancer Epidemiology, Biomarkers and Prevention* 13 (2004):1665; John Robbins, *The Food Revolution: How Your Diet Can Help Save Your Life and the World* (Berkeley, CA: Conari Press, 2001). See also Caldwell B. Esselstyn, *Prevent and Reverse Heart Disease: The Revolutionary, Scientifically Proven, Nutrition-Based Cure* (New York: Penguin, 2008).

80 G. A. Colditz, et al., "Relation of Meat, Fat, and Fiber Intake to the Risk of Colon Cancer in a Prospective Study Among Women," *New England Journal of Medicine* 323.24 (13 Dec. 1990): 1664–1672; Madeline Vann, "High Meat Consumption Linked to Heightened Cancer Risk," *U.S. News & World Report,* 11 Dec. 2007, available at *http://health.usnews.com/usnews/ health/healthday/071211/high-meat-consumption-linked-to- heightened-cancer-risk.htm* (accessed 27 Mar. 2009).

81 See H. Araki, et al., "High-Risk Group for Benign Prostatic Hypertrophy," *Prostate* 4. 3 (1983): 253–264, *http://www .ncbi.nlm.nih.gov/pubmed/6189108* (accessed 27 Mar. 2009).

82 In *The Genocidal Mentality: Nazi Holocaust and Nuclear Threat* (New York: Basic Books, 1990), Robert Jay Lifton and Eric Markusen use these terms to describe professionals who support nuclear development. Robert Jay Lifton and Eric Markusen, *The Genocidal Mentality: Nazi Holocaust and Nuclear Threat,* (New York: Basic Books, 1990).

83 Ibid.

84 Information on the ADA's Corporate Sponsorship Program is available at *http://www.eatright.org/cps/rde/xchg/ada/hs.xsl/ home_10016_ENU_HTML.htm*

85 Robert Jay Lifton, *The Nazi Doctors: Medical Killing and the Psy- chology of Genocide* (New York: Basic Books, 1986); Lifton and Markusen.

86 For more information on the meat-masculinity connection, see Fiddes. Also see Adams and Donovan, and Adams, *The Sexual Politics of Meat.*

87 Physicians Committee for Responsible Medicine, "The Protein Myth," *http://www.pcrm.org/health/veginfo/vsk/protein_myth .html* (accessed 26 Mar. 2009).

88 Lifton, *The Nazi Doctors*; Lifton and Markusen.

89 Farb and Armelagos.

90 For information on morality and disgust, see works cited in the bibliography by Rozin et al. Also see Andras Angyal, "Disgust and Related Aversions," *Journal of Abnormal and Social Psychology*

36 (1941): 393–412; Michael Lemonick, "Why We Get Disgusted," *Time,* 24 May 2007, available at *http://www.time.com/time/magazine/article/0,9171,1625167,00.html* (26 Mar. 2009); Simone Schnall, Jonathan Haidt, and Gerald L. Clore, "Disgust as Embodied Moral Judgment," *Personality and Social Psychology Bulletin* 34.8 (2008): 1096–1109; Trine Tsouderos, "Some Facial Expressions Are Part of a Primal 'Disgust Response,' University of Toronto Study Finds," *Chicago Tribune,* 27 Feb. 2009, available at *http://www.chicagotribune.com/news/nationworld/chi-talk-disgust-27feb27,0,5822692.story* (accessed 26 Mar. 2009); and Thalia Wheatley and Jonathon Haidt, "Hypnotically Induced Disgust Makes Moral Judgments More Severe," *Psychological Science* 16 (2005): 780–784.

91 Tsouderos.

92 Simoons, 106.

93 Farb and Armelagos, 167.

94 Kathy Berghorn, "Emily the Sacred Cow: Lewis Has Asked Me to Put Down Some of My Thoughts on Emily," 2 Apr. 2003, *http://www.peaceabbey.org/sanctuary/emily.htm#kathy* (accessed 2 July 2008).

95 Judith Herman, *Trauma and Recovery: The Aftermath of Violence—From Domestic Abuse to Political Terror* (New York: Basic Books, 1997), 1.

96 Sandra Blakeslee, "Cells That Read Minds," *The New York Times,* 10 Jan. 2006, available at *http://www.nytimes.com/2006/01/10/science/10mirr.html?pagewanted=3&_r=1&incamp=article_popular_2* (accessed 26 Mar. 2009); V. S. Ramachandran, "Mirror Neurons and the Brain in the Vat," *Edge: The Third Culture,* 10 Jan. 2006, available at *http://www.edge.org/3rd_culture/ramachandran06/ramachandran06_index.html*; (accessed 26 Mar. 2009); and "Children Are Naturally Prone to Be Empathic and Moral," *Science Daily,* 12 July 2008, available at *http://www.sciencedaily.com/releases/2008/07/080711080957.htm* (accessed 27 Mar. 2009).

97 From *The Witness,* James LaVeck, producer, and Jenny Stein, director, 2000.

98 Cited in Charles Patterson, *Eternal Treblinka: Our Treatment of Animals and the Holocaust* (New York: Lantern Books, 2002), 231.

99 Matthew Scully, *Dominion: The Power of Man, the Suffering of Animals, and the Call to Mercy* (New York: St. Martin's Press, 2002), 394.

100 All information in this paragraph is from the Union of Concerned Scientists, *http://www.ucsusa.org,* 1 Sep. 2008. See also notes from chapter 4.

101 James O'Dea, "Witnessing: A Form of Compassion," 2 Mar. 2007, *http://tow.charityfocus.org/?tid=502* (accessed 2 July 2008).

102 Cited in Patterson, 137.

103 Herman, 247.

BIBLIOGRAPHY

Adams, Carol J. "Feeding on Grace: Institutional Violence, Christianity, and Vegetarianism." In *Good News for Animals? Christian Approaches to Animal Well-Being,* edited by C. Pinches and J. B. McDaniel, 143–159. Maryknoll, NY: Orbis, 1993.

———. *Living Among Meat Eaters: The Vegetarian's Survival Handbook.* New York: Three Rivers Press, 2001.

———. *Neither Man nor Beast: Feminism and the Defense of Animals.* New York: Continuum, 1995.

———. *The Sexual Politics of Meat: A Feminist-Vegetarian Critical Theory.* New York: Continuum, 1992.

Adams, Carol J., and Josephine Donovan, eds. *Animals and Women: Feminist Theoretical Explorations.* Durham, NC: Duke University Press, 1995.

Allen, Michael, et al. "Values and Beliefs of Vegetarians and Omnivores." *Journal of Social Psychology* 140.4 (2000): 405–422.

Allport, Gordon. *The Nature of Prejudice.* New York: Addison-Wesley, 1958.

American Veterinary Medical Association. "Welfare Implications of the Veal Calf Husbandry." 13 Oct. 2008. *http://www.avma.org/issues/animal_welfare/veal_calf_husbandry_bgnd.asp* (accessed 27 Mar. 2009).

Anand, K. J. S., D. Phil, and P. R. Hickey. "Pain and Its Effects in the Human Neonate and Fetus." *New England Journal of Medicine* 317. 21. (Nov. 1987: 1321–1329. *http://www.cirp.org/library/pain/anand/* [accessed 27 Mar. 2009]).

———. *CIRP.org:* The Circumcision Reference Library. 5 Sept. 2006. *http://www.cirp.org/library/pain/anand/.*

Angyal, Andras. "Disgust and Related Aversions." *Journal of Abnormal and Social Psychology* 36 (1941): 393–412.

"Animal Cruelty Laws Among Fastest-Growing." *MSNBC.* 15 Feb. 2009. *http://www.msnbc.msn.com/id/29180079/* (accessed 26 Mar. 2009).

Araki, H., et al. "High-Risk Group for Benign Prostatic Hypertrophy." *Prostate* 4. 3 (1983): 253–264. *http://www.ncbi.nlm.nih .gov/pubmed/6189108* (accessed 27 Mar. 2009).

————. *PubMed. http://www.ncbi.nlm.nih.gov/pubmed/6189108* (accessed 27 Mar. 2009).

Arluke, Arnold. "Uneasiness Among Laboratory Technicians." *Lab Animal* 19.4 (1990): 20–39.

Arluke, Arnold, and Frederic Hafferty. "From Apprehension to Fascination with 'Dog Lab': The Use of Absolutions by Medical Students." *Journal of Contemporary Ethnography* 25.2 (1996): 201–225.

Arluke, Arnold, and Clinton Sanders. *Regarding Animals.* Philadelphia: Temple University Press, 1996.

Aronson, Elliot. "Back to the Future: Retrospective Review of Leon Festinger's A Theory of Cognitive Dissonance." *American Journal of Psychology* 110 (1997): 127–137.

————. "Dissonance, Hypocrisy, and the Self-Concept." In *Cognitive Dissonance: Progress on A Pivotal Theory in Social Psychology,* edited by E. Harmon-Jones and J. Mills, 103–126. Washington, DC: American Psychological Association, 1999.

Ascherio, Alberto, Graham A. Colditz, Edward Giovannucci, Eric B. Rimm, Meir J. Stampfer, and Walter C. Willett. "Intake of Fat, Meat, and Fiber in Relation to Risk of Colon Cancer in Men." *Cancer Research* 54 (1994): 2390–2397.

Augoustinos, Martha, and Katherine Reynolds, eds. *Understanding Prejudice, Racism, and Social Conflict.* Thousand Oaks, CA: Sage Publications, 2001.

Austin, Liz. "Whole Foods Bans Sale of Live Lobsters." *CBSnews.com.* 16 June 2006. *http://www.cbsnews.com/stories/2006/06/16/ap/ business/mainD8199PROO.shtml* (accessed 27 Mar. 2009).

Barrows, Anita. "The Ecopsychology of Child Development." In *Ecopsychology: Restoring the Earth, Healing the Mind,* edited by T. Roszak, M. E. Gomes, and D. Kanner, 101–110. San Francisco: Sierra Club Books, 1995.

Barthes, Roland. "Toward a Psychosociology of Contemporary Food Consumption." In *Food and Drink in History: Selections from the Annales Economies, Societes, Civilisations: Vol. 5,* edited by Robert Forster and Orest Ranum, 166–173. Baltimore and London: Johns Hopkins University Press, 1979.

Beardsworth, Alan, and Teresa Keil. "Contemporary Vegetarianism in the U.K.: Challenge and Incorporation?" *Appetite* 20 (1993): 229–234.

————. "The Vegetarian Option: Varieties, Conversions, Motives and Careers." *The Sociological Review* 40 (1992): 253–293.

Belasco, Warren. "Food, Morality, and Social Reform." In *Morality and Health,* edited by Allen Brandt and Paul Rozin, 185–199. New York: Rutledge, 1997.

Bell, A. Chris, et al. "A Method for Describing Food Beliefs Which May Predict Personal Food Choice." *Journal of Nutrition Education* 13.1 (1981): 22–26.

Bhatnagar, Parija. "PETA's Impotence Ad a No-No with CBS." CNN. 15 Jan. 2004. *http://money.cnn.com/2004/01/15/news/ companies/peta_cbssuperbowl/index.htm* (accessed 27 Mar. 2009).

Biermann-Ratjen, Eva Maria. "Incongruence and Psychopathology." In *Person-Centered Therapy: A European Perspective,* edited by B. Thorne and E. Lambers, 119–130. London: Sage Publications, 1998.

Bittman, Julie Cart, "Land Study on Grazing Denounced," *Los Angeles Times,* 18 June 2005. *http://articles.latimes.com/2005/jun/18/ nation/na-grazing18* (accessed 26 Mar. 2009).

Bittman, Mark. "Rethinking the Meat-Guzzler." *The New York Times.* 27 Jan. 2008. *http://www.nytimes.com/2008/01/27/ weekinreview/27bittman.html?_r=2* (accessed 26 Mar. 2009).

————. "Cells That Read Minds." *The New York Times.* 10 Jan. 2006. *http://www.nytimes.com/2006/01/10/science/10mirr. html?pagewanted=3&_r=1&incamp=article_popular_2* (accessed 26 Mar. 2009).

Blakeslee, Sandra. "Minds of Their Own: Birds Gain Rspect." *The New York Times.* 1 Feb. 2005. *http://www.nytimes.com/2005/ 02/01/science/01bird.html* (accessed 31 Mar. 2009).

Boat, Barbara. "The Relationship Between Violence to Children and Violence to Animals: An Ignored Link?" *Journal of Interpersonal Violence* 10.2 (1995): 228–235.

Booth, David. *The Psychology of Nutrition.* Bristol, PA: Taylor & Francis, 1994.

Brown, Culum, Kevin Laland, and Jens Krause, eds. *Fish Cognition and Behavior.* Oxford, UK: Blackwell Publishing, 2006.

Brown, Lesley Melville. *Cruelty to Animals: The Moral Debt.* London: Macmillan Press, 1988.

Calkins, A. "Observations on Vegetarian Dietary Practice and Social Factors: The Need for Further Research." *Perspectives in Practice* 74 (1979): 353–355.

Campbell, T. Colin, and Thomas M. Campell. *The China Study: The Most Comprehensive Study of Nutrition Ever Conducted and the Startling Implications for Diet, Weight Loss and Long-Term Health.* Dallas: Benbella Books, 2006.

Cart, Julie. "Land Study on Grazing Denounced." *Los Angeles Times* 18 June 2005. *http://articles.latimes.com/2005/jun/18/nation/ na-grazing18* (accessed 26 Mar. 2009).

Center for Responsive Politics. "Money in Politics—See Who's Giving and Who's Getting." *http://www.opensecrets.org/index.php* (accessed 25 Mar. 2009).

Center for Science in the Public Interest (CSPI). *http://www.cspinet .org/.*

Chamberlain, David B. "Babies Remember Pain." *CIRP.org:* The Circumcision Reference Library. 15 Dec. 2006. *http://www .cirp.org/library/psych/chamberlain/* (accessed 27 Mar. 2009).

————."Babies Remember Pain." *Journal of Prenatal and Perinatal Psychology and Health* 3. 4 (1989): 297–310. *http://www.cirp .org/library/psych/chamberlain* (accessed 27 Mar. 2009).

Chambers, J. P., et al. "Self-Selection of the Analgesic Drug Carprofen by Lame Broiler Chickens." *The Veterinary Record* 146.11 (2000): 307–311.

Chambers, P. G., et al. "Slaughter of Livestock." Food and Agriculture Organization of the United Nations. Apr. 2001. *http:// www.fao.org/docrep/003/x6909e/x6909e09.htm* (accessed 26 Mar. 2009).

"Children Are Naturally Prone to Be Empathic and Moral." *Science Daily.* 12 July 2008. *http://www.sciencedaily.com/ releases/2008/07/080711080957.htm* (accessed 27 Mar. 2009).

Chong, Jia-rui. "Wood-Chipped Chickens Fuel Outrage." *Los Angeles Times.* 22 Nov. 2003. *http://articles.latimes.com/2003/nov/22/ local/me-chipper22* (accessed 26 Mar. 2009).

Clarke, Paul, and Andrew Linzey. *Political Theory and Animal Rights.* Winchester, MA: Pluto Press, 1990.

Colditz, G. A., et al. "Relation of Meat, Fat, and Fiber Intake to the Risk of Colon Cancer in a Prospective Study Among Women." *New England Journal of Medicine* 323.24 (13 Dec. 1990): 1664–1672.

Compa, Lance, and Jamie Fellner. "Meatpacking's Human Toll." *The Washington Post.* 3 Aug. 2005. *http://www.washingtonpost.com/ wp-dyn/content/article/2005/08/02/AR2005080201936.html* (accessed 27 Mar. 2009).

Comstock, Gary L. "Pigs and Piety: A Theocentric Perspective on Food Animals." In *Good News for Animals? Christian Approaches to Animal Well-Being,* edited by Charles Pinches and Jay B. McDaniel, 105–127. Maryknoll, NY: Orbis, 1993.

Cone, Tracie. "Dairy Cows Head for Slaughter as Milk Prices Sour." Associated Press. 16 Feb. 2009. *http://www3 .signonsandiego.com/stories/2009/feb/16/farm-scene-cow-slaughter-021609/?zIndex=53727* (accessed 26 Mar. 2009).

Conrad, Peter, and Joseph Schneider. *Deviance and Medicalization: From Badness to Sickness.* Toronto: C.V. Mosby & Co., 1980.

Cooper, Charles, Thomas Wise, and Lee Mann. "Psychological and Cognitive Characteristics of Vegetarians." *Psychosomatics* 26.6 (1985): 521–527.

Counihan, Carol M. "Food Rules in the United States: Individualism, Control, and Hierarchy." *Anthropological Quarterly* 65 (1992): 55–66.

Davis, Karen. "Thinking Like a Chicken: Farm Animals and the Feminine Connection." In *Animals and Women: Feminist Theoretical Explorations,* edited by Carol J. Adams and Josephine Donovan, 192–212. Durham, NC: Duke University Press, 1995.

Dawn, Karen. *Thanking the Monkey: Rethinking the Way We Treat Animals.* New York: Harper, 2008.

Descartes, Rene. *A Discourse on the Method (Oxford World's Classics).* Trans. Ian Maclean. New York: Oxford University Press, 2006.

Devine, Tom. "Shielding the Giant: USDA's 'Don't Look, Don't Know' Policy for Beef Inspection." *WhistleBlower.org. http:// www.whistleblower.org/doc/S/Shielding%20the%20Giant%20 Final%20PDF.pdf* (accessed 27 Mar. 2009).

Dietz, Thomas, et al. "Social Psychological and Structural Influences on Vegetarian Beliefs." *Rural Sociology* 64.3 (1999): 500–511.

———, et al. "Values and Vegetarianism: An Exploratory Analysis." *Rural Sociology* 60.3 (1995): 533–542.

Dilanian, Ken. "Bill Includes Billions in Farm Subsidies." *USA Today.* 15 May 2008. *http://www.usatoday.com/news/washington/ 2008-05-15-farmbill_N.htm* (accessed 25 Mar. 2009).

Donaldson, Tammy McCormick. "Is Boredom Driving Pigs Crazy?" Working paper, the University of Idaho College of Natural

Resources. *http://www.cnr.uidaho.edu/range556/Appl_BEHAVE/projects/pigs_ster.html* (accessed 26 Mar. 2009).

Douglas, Mary. *Implicit Meanings: Essays in Anthropology.* London: Routledge & Kegan Paul, 1975.

Draycott, Simon, and Alan Dabbs. "Cognitive Dissonance: An Overview of the Literature and Its Integration into Theory and Practice in Clinical Psychology." *British Journal of Clinical Psychology* 37 (1998): 341–353.

Du, Wayne. "Porcine Stress Syndrome Gene and Pork Production." Ontario Ministry of Agriculture Food and Rural Affairs. June 2004. *http://www.omafra.gov.on.ca/english/livestock/swine/facts/04-053.htm* (accessed 27 Mar. 2009).

Dunayer, Joan. *Animal Equality: Language and Liberation.* Derwood, MD: Ryce Publishing, 2001.

Eisler, Riane. *The Chalice and the Blade: Our History, Our Future.* New York: HarperCollins, 1987.

Eisnitz, Gail. *Slaughterhouse: The Shocking Story of Greed, Neglect, and Inhumane Treatment Inside the U.S. Meat Industry.* Amherst, NY: Prometheus Books, 1997.

Esselstyn, Caldwell B. *Prevent and Reverse Heart Disease: The Revolutionary, Scientifically Proven, Nutrition-Based Cure.* New York: Penguin, 2008.

Ewers, Justin. "Don't Read This Over Dinner." *U.S. News and World Report.* 7 Aug. 2005. *http://www.usnews.com/usnews/culture/articles/050815/15meat.htm* (accessed 31 Mar. 2009).

"EWG Farm Bill 2007 Policy Analysis Database." *Environmental Working Group. http://farm.ewg.org/sites/farmbill2007/* (accessed 25 Mar. 2009).

Farb, Peter, and George Armelagos. *Consuming Passions: The Anthropology of Eating.* Boston: Houghton Mifflin, 1980.

Feldman, Megan. "Swift Meat Packing Plant and Illegal Immigrants." *The Houston Press.* 4 Apr. 2007. *http://www.houstonpress.com/2007-04-05/news/swift-meatpacking-plant-and-illegal-immigrants/* (accessed 27 Mar. 2009).

Fessler, Daniel M. T., and Carlos David Navarrette. "Meat Is Good to Taboo: Dietary Proscriptions as a Product of the Interaction of Psychological Mechanisms and Social Processes." *Journal of Cognition and Culture* 3. 1 (2003): 1–40. *http://www.sscnet.ucla.edu/anthro/faculty/fessler/pubs/MeatIsGoodToTaboo.pdf* (accessed 26 Mar. 2009).

————. UCLA. *http://www.sscnet.ucla.edu/anthro/faculty/fessler/pubs/MeatIsGoodToTaboo.pdf* (accessed 26 Mar. 2009).

Festinger, Leon. *A Theory of Cognitive Dissonance.* Evanston, IL: Row, Peterson, 1957.

Fiddes, Nick. *Meat: A Natural Symbol.* New York: Rutledge, 1991.

Finsen, Lawrence, and Susan Finsen. *The Animal Rights Movement in America: From Compassion to Respect.* New York: Twayne Publishers, 1994.

Fischler, Claude. "Food Habits, Social Change and the Nature/Culture Dilemma." *Social Science Information* 19.6 (1980): 937–953.

————. "Food, Self and Identity." *Social Science Information.* 27.2 (1988): 275–292.

"Fish May Actually Feel Pain and React to It Much Like Humans Do." *Science Daily.* 1 May 2009. *http://www.sciencedaily.com/releases/2009/04/090430161242.htm* (accessed 4 June 2009).

Food and Agriculture Organization of the United Nations. " Livestock's Long Shadow: Environmental Issues and Options." 2006. *http://www.fao.org/docrep/010/a0701e/a0701e00.htm* (accessed 27 Mar. 2009).

————. "Pro-Poor Livestock Policy Initiative." *http://www.fao.org/AG/AGAInfo/programmes/en/pplpi/docarc/pb_hpaibiosecurity.html* (accessed 26 Mar. 2009).

"Food Taboos: It's All a Matter of Taste." *National Geographic News.* 19 Apr. 2004. *http://news.nationalgeographic.com/news/2004/04/0419_040419_TVfoodtaboo.html* (accessed 26 Mar. 2009).

Fox, Michael Allen. *Deep Vegetarianism.* Philadelphia: Temple University Press, 1999.

Francione, Gary. *Animals, Property, and the Law.* Philadelphia: Temple University Press, 1995.

Friedman, Stanley. "On Vegetarianism." *Journal of the American Psychoanalytic Association* 23.2 (1975): 396–406.

Frommer, Frederic J. "Video Shows Workers Abusing Pigs." *The Guardian Unlimited.* 17 Sep. 2008. *http://www.guardian.co.uk/uslatest/story/0,,-7805670,00.html* (accessed 31 Mar. 2009).

Furst, Tanis, et al. "Food Choice: A Conceptual Model of the Process." *Appetite* 26 (1996): 247–266.

Garner, Robert, ed. *Animal Rights: The Changing Debate.* New York: New York University Press, 1996.

Gaudette, Karen. "USDA Expands Ground-Beef Recall." *The Seattle Times.* 4 July 2008. *http://seattletimes.nwsource.com/html/nationworld/2008033109_beefrecall04.html* (accessed 27 Mar. 2009).

Gofton, L. "The Rules of the Table: Sociological Factors Influencing Food Choice." In *The Food Consumer,* by Christopher Ritson, Leslie Gofton, and John McKenzie, 127–153. New York: John Wiley & Sons, 1986.

Greger, Michael. *Bird Flu: A Virus of Our Own Hatching.* New York: Lantern Books, 2006.

Grossman, Dave. *On Killing: The Psychological Cost of Learning to Kill in War and Society.* New York: Back Bay Books, 1996.

Gurian-Sherman, Doug. "CAFOs Uncovered: The Untold Costs of Confined Animal Feeding Operations." Union of Concerned Scientists. Apr. 2008. *http://www.ucsusa.org/assets/documents/food_and_agriculture/cafos-uncovered-executive-summary.pdf* (accessed 31 Mar. 2009).

Halpin, Zuleyma Tang. "Scientific Objectivity and the Concept of the 'Other.'" *Women's Studies International Forum* 12.3 (1989): 285–294.

Hamilton, Malcolm. "Wholefoods and Healthfoods: Beliefs and Attitudes." *Appetite* 20 (1993): 223–228.

Harmon-Jones, Eddie, and Judson Mills, eds. *Cognitive Dissonance: Progress on a Pivotal Theory in Social Psychology.* Washington, DC: American Psychological Association, 1999.

Hedges, Stephen J., and Washington Bureau. "E. Coli Loophole Cited in Recalls Tainted Meat Can Be Sold if Cooked." *Chicago Tribune.* 11 Nov. 2007. *http://archives.chicagotribune.com/2007/nov/11/food/chi-meat_bdnov11* (accessed 27 Mar. 2009).

————. "Topps Meat Recall Raises Questions About Inspections Workload." *Chicago Tribune.* 14 Oct. 2007. *http://archives. chicagotribune.com/2007/oct/14/food/chi-meat_5s_hedgesoct14* (accessed 27 Mar. 2009).

Heffernan, William, and Mary Hendrickson. "Concentration of Agricultural Markets." *National Farmer's Union.* Apr. 2007. *http://www.nfu.org/wp-content/2007-heffernanreport.pdf* (accessed 25 Mar. 2009).

Hegeman, Roxana. "Injuries Propel Union's Offences." *Arkansas Democrat Gazette.* 18 Feb. 2007. *http://www.nwanews.com/adg/Business/182284/* (accessed 27 Mar. 2009).

Herman, Judith. *Trauma and Recovery: The Aftermath of Violence—From Domestic Abuse to Political Terror.* New York: Basic Books, 1997.

Hindley, M. Patricia. "'Minding Animals': The Role of Animals in Children's Mental Development." In *Attitudes to Animals: Views in Animal Welfare,* edited by F. L. Dolins, 186–199. Cambridge, UK: Cambridge University Press, 1999.

Holm, Lotte, and M. Mohl. "The Role of Meat in Everyday Food Culture: An Analysis of an Interview Study in Copenhagen." *Appetite* 34 (2000): 277–283.

Howard, George S. *Ecological Psychology: Creating a More Earth-Friendly Human Nature.* Notre Dame, IN: University of Notre Dame Press, 1997.

Human Rights Watch. "Blood, Sweat and Fear." *HRW.org.* 24 Jan. 2005. *http://www.hrw.org/en/node/11869/section/5* (accessed 27 Mar. 2009).

Humane Society of the United States. "Undercover Investigation Reveals Rampant Animal Cruelty at California Slaughter Plant—A Major Beef Supplier to America's School Lunch Program." 30 Jan. 2008. *http://www.hsus.org/farm/news/ournews/undercover_investigation.html* (accessed 26 Mar. 2009).

Irvin, David. "Control Debate, Growers Advised." *Arkansas-Democrat Gazette,* Northwest Arkansas edition. 22 Sep. 2007. *http://www.nwanews.com/adg/Business/202171/* (accessed 26 Mar. 2009).

Jabs, Jennifer, Carol Devine, and J. Sobal. "Model of the Process of Adopting Vegetarian Diets: Health Vegetarians and Ethical Vegetarians." *Journal of Nutrition Education* 30.4 (1998): 196–202.

Jacobsen, Ken, and Linda Riebel. *Eating to Save the Earth: Food Choices for a Healthy Planet.* Berkeley, CA: Celestial Arts, 2002.

Johns Hopkins Bloomberg School of Public Health. "Public Health Association Calls for Moratorium on Factory Farms; Cites Health Issues, Pollution." 9 Jan. 2004. *http://www.jhsph.edu/publichealthnews/press_releases/PR_2004/farm_moratorium.html* (accessed 26 Mar. 2009).

Johnson, Allan G. *The Forest and the Trees: Sociology as Life, Practice and Promise.* Philadelphia: Temple University Press, 1997.

Joy, Melanie. "From Carnivore to Carnist: Liberating the Language of Meat." *Satya* 8.2 (2001): 26–27.

———. "Humanistic Psychology and Animal Rights: Reconsidering the Boundaries of the Humanistic Ethic." *Journal of Humanistic Psychology* 45.1 (2005): 106–130.

———. "Psychic Numbing and Meat Consumption: The Psychology of Carnism." Diss., Saybrook Graduate School, 2003.

———. *Strategic Action for Animals: A Handbook on Strategic Movement Building, Organizing, and Activism for Animal Liberation.* New York: Lantern Books, 2008.

Jung, C. G. "The Problem of Evil Today." In *Meeting the Shadow: The Hidden Power of the Dark Side of Human Nature,* edited by C. Zweig and J. Abrams, 170–173. New York: Putnam, 1991.

Kapleau, Philip. *To Cherish All Life: A Buddhist Case for Becoming Vegetarian*. Rochester, NY: The Zen Center, 1986.

Kellert, Stephen R., and Alan Felthous. "Childhood Cruelty Toward Animals Among Criminals and Noncriminals." *Human Relations* 38.12 (1985): 1113–1129.

Kelly, Daniel. "The Role of Psychology in the Study of Culture." Purdue University. *http://web.ics.purdue.edu/~drkelly/ KellyMacheryMallonMasonStichCommentonMesoudietal.htm* (accessed 26 Mar. 2009).

Kirby, Alex, "Fish Do Feel Pain, Scientists Say." *BBC News Online http://news.bbc.co.uk/2/hi/science/nature/2983045.stm* (accessed 4 June 2009).

Kowalski, Gary. *The Souls of Animals*. Walpole, NH: Stillpoint, 1991.

Lea, Emma, and Anthony Worsley. "Influences on Meat Consumption in Australia." *Appetite* 36 (2001): 127–136.

Lee, Jennifer. "Neighbors of Vast Hog Farms Say Foul Air Endangers Their Health." *The New York Times*. 11 May 2003. *http://www .nytimes.com/2003/05/11/us/neighbors-of-vast-hog-farms-say-foul-air-endangers-their-health.html* (accessed 26 Mar. 2009).

Lemonick, Michael. "Why We Get Disgusted." *Time*. 24 May 2007 *http://www.time.com/time/magazine/article/ 0,9171,1625167,00.html* (accessed 26 Mar. 2009).

Lifton, Robert Jay. "Beyond Psychic Numbing: A Call to Awareness." *American Journal of Orthopsychiatry* 52.4 (1982): 619–629.

————. *The Nazi Doctors: Medical Killing and the Psychology of Genocide*. New York: Basic Books, 1986.

————. "A Nuclear Age Ethos: Ten Psychological-Ethical Principles." *Journal of Humanistic Psychology* 25.4 (1985): 39–40.

Lifton, Robert Jay, and Eric Markusen. *The Genocidal Mentality: Nazi Holocaust and Nuclear Threat*. New York: Basic Books, 1990.

Lilliston, Ben. "A Fair Farm Bill for Competitive Markets." Institute for Agriculture and Trade Policy. 2007. *http://www.agobservatory .org/library.cfm?refid=98445* (accessed 29 Mar. 2009).

Lindeman, Marjaana, and M. Väänänen. "Measurement of Ethical Food Choice Motives." *Appetite* 34 (2000): 55–59.

LJ. "Stop the Dog Meat Industry." ASPCA Online Community. 18 Feb. 2009. *http://aspcacommunity.ning.com/forum/topics/stop-the-dog-meat-industry* (accessed 26 Mar. 2009).

Lobo, Phillip. "Animal Welfare and Activism: What You Need to Know." PowerPoint presentation at the FMI-AMI Meat Conference. 10 Mar. 2008. *http://www.meatconference.com/ht/a/GetDocumentAction/i/38151* (accessed 26 Mar. 2009).

Locatelli, Margaret Garrett, and Robert Holt. "Antinuclear Activism, Psychic Numbing, and Mental Health." *International Journal of Mental Health* 15.1–3 (1986): 143–161.

Lovelock, James. *Gaia: A New Look at Life on Earth.* Oxford, UK: Oxford University Press, 1979.

Macy, Joanna. "Working Through Environmental Despair." In *Ecopsychology: Restoring the Earth, Healing the Mind,* edited by T. Roszak, M. E. Gomes, and A. D. Kanner, 240–259. San Francisco: Sierra Club Books, 1995.

Marcus, Erik. *Meat Market: Animals, Ethics, and Money.* Ithaca, NY: Brio Press, 2005.

———. *Vegan: The New Ethics of Eating.* Ithaca, NY: McBooks, 1998.

Maslow, Abraham. *Motivation and Personality.* 3rd ed. New York: Harper & Row, 1987.

Masson, Jeffrey. *The Face on Your Plate: The Truth About Food.* New York: W. W. Norton, 2009.

Mattera, Philip. "USDA Inc.: How Agribusiness Has Hijacked Regulatory Policy at the U.S. Department of Agriculture." Corporate research project of Good Jobs First. 23 July 2004. *http://www.agribusinessaccountability.org/pdfs/289_USDAInc..pdf* (accessed 25 Mar. 2009).

Mattes, Richard D. "Learned Food Aversions: A Family Study." *Physiology and Behavior* 50 (1991): 499–504.

Maurer, Donna. *Vegetarianism: Movement or Moment?* Philadelphia: Temple University Press, 2002.

McDonald, Barbara, Ronald M. Cervero, and Bradley C. Courtenay. "An Ecological Perspective of Power in Transformational Learning: A Case Study of Ethical Vegans." *Adult Education Quarterly* 50.1 (1999): 5–23.

McDougall, John A., and Mary McDougall. *The McDougall Program: Twelve Days to Dynamic Health.* New York: Plume, 1991.

McElroy, Damien. "Korean Outrage as West Tries to Use World Cup to Ban Dog Eating." *Telegraph.* 6 Jan. 2002. *http://www.telegraph. co.uk/news/worldnews/europe/france/1380569/Korean-outrage-as-West-tries-to-use-World-Cup-to-ban-dog-eating.html* (accessed 26 Mar. 2009).

Messina, Virginia, and Mark Messina. *The Vegetarian Way.* New York: Crown Trade Paperbacks, 1996.

Metzner, Ralph. *Green Psychology: Transforming Our Relationship to the Earth.* Rochester, VT: Park Street Press, 1999.

Midei, Aimee. "Identification of the First Gene in Posttraumatic Stress Disorder." *Bio-Medicine.* 22 Sep. 2002. *http://news. bio-medicine.org/biology-news-2/Identification-of-the-first-gene-in-posttraumatic-stress-disorder-6692-1/* (accessed 27 Mar. 2009).

Midgley, Mary. *Animals and Why They Matter: A Journey Around the Species Barrier.* New York: Penguin, 1983.

Milgram, Stanley. *Obedience to Authority: An Experimental View.* New York: Harper & Row, 1974.

Mintz, Sidney. *Tasting Food, Tasting Freedom: Excursions into Eating, Culture, and the Past.* Boston: Beacon Press, 1996.

Mitchell, C. E. "Animals—Sacred or Secondary? Ideological Influences on Therapist and Client Priorities and Approaches to Decision-Making." *Psychology* 30.1 (1993): 22–28.

Mittal, Anuradha. "Giving Away the Farm: The 2002 Farm Bill." The Oakland Institute. June 2002. *http://www.oaklandinstitute. org/?q=node/view/39* (accessed 27 Mar. 2009). The Oakland Institute is a policy think tank whose focus is on increasing public participation in, and fair debate on, critical social and environmental issues. Anuradha Mittal (the institute's executive director) was named most valuable thinker of 2008 by *Nation* magazine.

"More Urban, Suburban Homes Have Pet Chickens." *Dallas Morning News*. 16 July 2007. *http://www.dallasnews.com/sharedcontent/ dws/news/localnews/stories/071707dnmetpetchickens.ca7efd.html* (accessed 27 Mar. 2009).

Morgan, Dan, Gilbert M. Gaul, and Sarah Cohen. "Harvesting Cash: A Year-Long Investigation into Farm Subsidies." *The Washington Post*. 2006. *http://www.washingtonpost.com/wp-srv/nation/ interactives/farmaid/* (accessed 25 Mar. 2009).

Morrow, Julie. "An Overview of Current Dairy Welfare Concerns from the North American Perspective." 19 Dec. 2002. *http:// www.nal.usda.gov/awic/pubs/dairy/overview.htm* (accessed 27 Mar. 2009).

Motovalli, Jim. "The Meat of the Matter: Our Livestock Industry Creates More Greenhouse Gas Than Transportation Does." *E Magazine* 19.4 (July/Aug. 2008).

Murcott, A. "You Are What You Eat: Anthropological Factors Influencing Food Choice." In *The Food Consumer*, edited by Christopher Ritson, Leslie Gofton, and John McKenzie, 107–125. New York: John Wiley & Sons, 1986.

National Endowment for the Humanities. "Voting Rights for Women: Pro- and Anti- Suffrage." *EDSITEment.com*. 11 June 2002. *http://edsitement.neh.gov/view_lesson_plan.asp?id=438* (accessed 27 Mar. 2009).

National Resources Defense Council. "Pollution from Giant Livestock Farms Threatens Public Health." 15 July 2005. *http://www.nrdc. org/water/pollution/nspills.asp* (accessed 26 Mar. 2009).

"Nebraska Beef Recalls 1.2 Million Pounds of Beef." *MSNBC.com*. 10 Aug. 2008. *http://www.msnbc.msn.com/id/26101733/* (accessed 27 Mar. 2009).

Nestle, Marion. *Food Politics: How the Food Industry Influences Nutrition and Health*. Berkeley: University of California Press, 2007.

Nibert, David Allen. *Animal Rights/Human Rights: Entanglements of Oppression and Liberation*. Lanham, MD: Rowman & Littlefield, 2002.

Norberg-Hodge, Helena. "Compassion in the Age of the Global Economy." *The Psychology of Awakening: Buddhism, Science, and Our Day-to-Day Lives,* edited by G. Watson, S. Batchelor, and G. Claxton, 55–67. York Beach, ME: Samuel Weiser, 2000.

Passariello, Phyllis. "Me and My Totem: Cross-Cultural Attitudes Towards Animals." *Attitudes to Animals: Views in Animal Welfare,* edited by F. L. Dolins, 12–25. Cambridge, UK: Cambridge University Press, 1999.

Patterson, Charles. *Eternal Treblinka: Our Treatment of Animals and the Holocaust.* New York: Lantern Books, 2002.

Petrinovich, L., P. O'Neill, and M. Jorgensen. "An Empirical Study of Moral Intuition: Toward an Evolutionary Ethics." *Journal of Personality and Social Psychology* 64.3 (1993): 467–478.

Phillips, Mary T. "Savages, Drunks, and Lab Animals: The Researcher's Perception of Pain." *Society and Animals* 1.1 (1993): 61–81.

Phillips, R. L. "Coronary Heart Disease Mortality Among Seventh Day Adventists with Differing Dietary Habits; a Preliminary Report." *Cancer Epidemiology, Biomarkers and Prevention* 13 (2004): 1665.

Physicians Committee for Responsible Medicine. "The Protein Myth." *http://www.pcrm.org/health/veginfo/vsk/protein_myth.html* (accessed 26 Mar. 2009).

Pickert, Kate. "Undercover Animal-Rights Investigator" *Time.* 9 Mar. 2009. *http://www.time.com/time/nation/article/0,8599,1883742,00.html* (accessed 26 Mar. 2009).

Pilisuk, Marc. "Cognitive Balance and Self-Relevant Attitudes." *Journal of Abnormal and Social Psychology* 6.2 (1962): 95–103.

———. "The Hidden Structure of Contemporary Violence." *Peace and Conflict: Journal of Peace Psychology* 4 (1998): 197–216.

Pilisuk, Marc, and Melanie Joy. "Humanistic Psychology and Ecology." *The Handbook of Humanistic Psychology: Leading Edges in Theory, Research and Practice,* edited by K. J. Schneider, J. T. Bugental, and J. F. Pierson, 101–114. Thousand Oaks, CA: Sage Publications, 2000.

Plous, Scott. "Psychological Mechanisms in the Human Use of Animals." *Journal of Social Issues* 49.1 (1993): 11–52.

Pollan, Michael. *The Omnivore's Dilemma: A Natural History of Four Meals.* New York: Penguin, 2006.

———. "Power Steer." *The New York Times.* 31 Mar. 2002, sec. 6.

Prilleltensky, Isaac. "Psychology and the Status Quo." *American Psychologist* 44.5 (1989): 795–802.

Public Broadcasting Service (PBS). "Meatpacking in the U.S.: Still a 'Jungle' Out There?" Episode description for the news program *NOW.* 15 Dec. 2006. *http://www.pbs.org/now/shows/250/ meat-packing.html* (accessed 26 Mar. 2009).

Ramachandran, V. S. "Mirror Neurons and the Brain in the Vat." *Edge: The Third Culture.* 10 Jan. 2006. *http://www.edge.org/3rd_ culture/ramachandran06/ramachandran06_index.html* (accessed 26 Mar. 2009).

Randour, Mary Lou. *Animal Grace: Entering a Spiritual Relationship with Our Fellow Creatures.* Novato, CA: New World Library, 2000.

Regan, Tom. *The Case for Animal Rights.* Berkeley: University of California Press, 1983.

"Retailer Recalls Parkas Trimmed in Dog Fur." *The New York Times.* 16 Dec. 1998. *http://www.nytimes.com/1998/12/16/nyregion/ retailer-recalls-parkas-trimmed-in-dog-fur.html?n=Top/News/ Science/Topics/Dogs* (accessed 27 Mar. 2009).

Richardson, N. J. "UK Consumer Perceptions of Meat." *Proceedings of the Nutrition Society* 53 (1994): 281–287.

Richardson, N. J., R. Shepard, and N. A. Elliman. "Current Attitudes and Future Influences on Meat Consumption in the U.K." *Appetite* 21 (1993): 41–51.

Rifkin, Jeremy. *Beyond Beef: The Rise and Fall of the Cattle Culture.* New York: Plume, 1992.

Robbins, John. *Diet for a New America.* Tiburon, CA: H. J. Kramer, 1987.

———. *The Food Revolution: How Your Diet Can Help Save Your Life and the World.* Berkeley, CA: Conari Press, 2001.

Rogers, Carl. *On Becoming a Person.* Boston: Houghton Mifflin, 1961.

"Role of the Meat and Poultry Industry in the U.S. Economy." *American Meat Institute.* 2000. *http://www.meatami.com//content/ PressCenter/FactSheets_InfoKits/Intl_trade_kit.htm* (accessed 1 Nov. 2001).

Rosen, Steven. *Diet for Transcendence: Vegetarianism and the World Religions.* Badger, CA: Torchlight Publishing, 1997.

Rostler, Suzanne. "Vegetarian Diet May Mask Eating Disorder in Teens." *Journal of Adolescent Health* 29 (2001): 406–416.

Rozin, Paul. "Moralization." In *Morality and Health,* edited by A. Brandt and P. Rozin, 379–401. New York: Rutledge, 1997.

———. "A Perspective on Disgust." *Psychological Review* 94.1 (1987): 23–41.

Rozin, Paul, and April Fallon. "The Psychological Categorization of Foods and Non-Foods: A Preliminary Taxonomy of Food Rejections." *Appetite* 1 (1980): 193–201.

Rozin, Paul, Maureen Markwith, and Caryn Stoess. "Moralization and Becoming a Vegetarian: The Transformation of Preferences into Values and the Recruitment of Disgust." *Psychological Science* 8.2 (1977): 67–73.

Rozin, Paul, M. L. Pelchat, and A. E. Fallon. "Psychological Factors Influencing Food Choice." In *The Food Consumer,* edited by C. Ritson, L. Gofton, and J. McKenzie, 85–106. New York: John Wiley & Sons, 1986.

Ryder, Richard D. *The Political Animal: The Conquest of Speciesism.* Jefferson, NC: McFarland & Company, 1998.

Sapp, Stephen G., and Wendy J. Harrod. "Social Acceptability and Intentions to Eat Beef: An Expansion of the Fishbein-Ajzen Model Using Reference Group Theory." *Rural Sociology* 54.3 (1989): 420–438.

Schafer, Robert, and Elizabeth A. Yetley. "Social Psychology of Food Faddism." *Journal of the American Dietetic Association* 66 (1975): 129–133.

Schlosser, Eric. "The Chain Never Stops." *Mother Jones.* July/Aug. 2001. *http://www.motherjones.com/news/feature/2001/07/ meatpacking.html* (accessed 27 Mar. 2009).

————. "Fast Food Nation: Meat and Potatoes." *Rolling Stone.* 3 Sep. 1998. *http://www.ericsecho.org/investigation2.htm.*

————. *Fast Food Nation: The Dark Side of the All-American Meal.* New York: Houghton Mifflin, 2001.

————. "Tyson's Moral Anchor." *The Nation.* 24 June 2004. *http:// www.thenation.com/doc/20040712/schlosser* (accessed 27 Mar. 2009).

Schnall, Simone, Jonathan Haidt, and Gerald L. Clore. "Disgust as Embodied Moral Judgment." *Personality and Social Psychology Bulletin* 34.8 (2008): 1096–1109.

Schwartz, Richard H. *Judaism and Vegetarianism.* New York: Lantern Books, 2001.

Scully, Matthew. *Dominion: The Power of Man, the Suffering of Animals, and the Call to Mercy.* New York: St. Martin's Griffin Press, 2002.

Serpell, James A. *In the Company of Animals.* New York: Basil Blackwell, 1986.

————. "Sheep in Wolves' Clothing? Attitudes to Animals Among Farmers and Scientists." In *Attitudes to Animals: Views in Animal Welfare,* edited F. L. Dolins, 26–33. Cambridge, UK: Cambridge University Press, 1999.

Severson, Kim. "Upton Sinclair, Now Playing on YouTube." *The New York Times.* 12 Mar. 2008. *http://www.nytimes.com/2008/03/12/ dining/12animal.html?pagewanted=1&_r=3* (accessed 26 Mar. 2009).

Shapiro, Kenneth J. "Animal Rights Versus Humanism: The Charge of Speciesism." *Journal of Humanistic Psychology* 30.2 (1990): 9–37.

Shepard, Paul. *The Tender Carnivore and the Sacred Game.* New York: Scribners, 1973.

Shickle, D., et al. "Differences in Health, Knowledge and Attitudes Between Vegetarians and Meat Eaters in a Random Population Sample." *Journal of the Royal Society of Medicine* 82 (1989): 18–20.

"Short Supply of Inspectors Threatens Meat Safety." *MSNBC.com.* 21 Feb. 2008. *http://www.msnbc.msn.com/id/23282496/* (accessed 27 Mar. 2009).

Simoons, Frederick J. *Eat Not This Flesh: Food Avoidances in the Old World.* Madison: University of Wisconsin Press, 1961.

Sims, L. S. "Food-Related Value-Orientations, Attitudes, and Beliefs of Vegetarians and Non-Vegetarians." *Ecology of Food and Nutrition* 7 (1978): 23–35.

Sinclair, Upton. *The Jungle.* New York: Penguin Classics, 2006.

Singer, Peter. *Animal Liberation.* New York: Avon Books, 1990.

Slovic, Paul. "'If I Look at the Mass I Will Never Act': Psychic Numbing and Genocide." *Judgment and Decision Making* 2.2 (2007): 79–95.

Smith, Allen C., and Sherryl Kleinman. "Managing Emotions in Medical School: Students' Contacts with the Living and the Dead." *Social Psychology Quarterly* 52.1 (1989): 56–69.

Sneddon, L.U., V. A. Braithwaite, and M. J. Gentle. "Do Fishes Have Nociceptors? Evidence for the Evolution of a Vertebrate Sensory System." *Proceedings of the Royal Society of London,* B 270. 1520 (7 June 2003): 1115–1121.

Spencer, Colin. *The Heretic's Feast: A History of Vegetarianism.* Hanover, NH: University Press of New England, 1995.

Spiegel, Marjorie. *The Dreaded Comparison: Human and Animal Slavery.* New York: Mirror Books, 1988.

Stamm, B. Hudnall, ed. *Secondary Traumatic Stress: Self-Care Issues for Clinicians, Researchers, and Educators.* 2nd ed. Baltimore, MD: Sidran Press, 1999.

Stepaniak, Joanne. *The Vegan Sourcebook.* Los Angeles: Lowell House, 1998.

Stout, Martha. *The Sociopath Next Door.* New York: Broadway Books, 2005.

Thich Nhat Hanh. *For a Future to Be Possible: Commentaries on the Five Wonderful Precepts.* Berkeley, CA: Parallax Press, 1993.

Tolle, Eckhart. *A New Earth: Awakening to Your Life's Purpose.* New York: Plume, 2005.

————. *The Power of Now: A Guide to Spiritual Enlightenment.* Novato, CA: New World Library, 1999.

Tsouderos, Trine. "Some Facial Expressions Are Part of a Primal 'Disgust Response', University of Toronto Study Finds." *Chicago Tribune.* 27 Feb. 2009. *http://www.chicagotribune.com/news/nationworld/chi-talk-disgust-27feb27,0,5822692.story* (accessed 26 Mar. 2009).

Twigg, Julia. "Vegetarianism and the Meanings of Meat." In *The Sociology of Food and Eating,* edited by A. Murcott, and A. Aldershot, 18–30. England: Gomer Publishing, 1983.

Union of Concerned Scientists. "Outbreak of a Resistant Food Borne Illness." 18 July 2003. *http://www.ucsusa.org/food_and_agriculture/science_and_impacts/impacts_industrial_agriculture/outbreak-of-a-resistant.html* (accessed 27 Mar. 2009).

————. "They Eat What? The Reality of Feed at Animal Factories." 8 Aug. 2006. *http://www.ucsusa.org/food_and_agriculture/science_and_impacts/impacts_industrial_agriculture/they-eat-what-the-reality-of.html* (accessed 27 Mar. 2009).

U.S. Department of Agriculture. "Nebraska Firm Recalls Beef Products Due to Possible E. coli O157:H7 Contamination." 30 June 2008. *http://www.fsis.usda.gov/News_&_Events/Recall_022_2008_Release/index.asp* (accessed 27 Mar. 2009).

U.S. Department of Agriculture, Grain Inspection, Packers, and Stockyards Administration (GIPSA). *http://www.gipsa.usda.gov/GIPSA/webapp?area=newsroom&subject=landing&topic=cc-budget-03* (accessed 30 Mar. 2009). Statement of David R. Shipman, acting administrator of the Grain Inspection, Packers, and Stockyards Administration, before the Subcommittee on Agriculture, Rural Development, and Related Agencies, in reference to the FY 2003 budget proposal.

U.S. Department of Labor. "Safety and Health Guide for the Meatpacking Industry." 1988. *http://www.osha.gov/Publications/OSHA3108/osha3108.html* (accessed 27 Mar. 2009).

Vann, Madeline. "High Meat Consumption Linked to Heightened Cancer Risk." *U.S. News & World Report.* 11 Dec. 2007. *http://health.usnews.com/usnews/health/healthday/071211/high-meat-consumption-linked-to-heightened-cancer-risk.htm* (accessed 27 Mar. 2009).

Vansickle, Joe. "Preparing Pigs for Transport." *The National Hog Farmer.* 15 Sep. 2008. *http://nationalhogfarmer.com/behavior-welfare/0915-preparing-pigs-transport/* (accessed 26 Mar. 2009).

Verhovek, Sam. "Gain for Winfrey in Suit by Beef Producers in Texas." *The New York Times.* 18 Feb. 1998. *http://query.nytimes.com/gst/fullpage.html?res=9407E0DE153FF93BA25751C0A96E958260&sec=health&spon=&pagewanted=1* (accessed 27 Mar. 2009).

Warrick, Joby. "They Die Piece by Piece." *The Washington Post.* 10 Apr. 2001. *http://www.hfa.org/hot_topic/wash_post.pdf* (accessed 26 Mar. 2009).

Weingarten, Kaethe. *Common Shock: Witnessing Violence Every Day.* New York: New American Library, 2004.

WGBH Educational Foundation. "Inside the Slaughterhouse." *http://www.pbs.org/wgbh/pages/frontline/shows/meat/slaughter/slaughterhouse.html* (accessed 27 Mar. 2009).

———. "What Is HAACP?" *http://www.pbs.org/wgbh/pages/frontline/shows/meat/evaluating/haacp.html* (accessed 27 Mar. 2009).

Wheatley, Thalia, and Jonathon Haidt. "Hypnotically Induced Disgust Makes Moral Judgments More Severe." *Psychological Science* 16 (2005): 780–784.

Wolf, David B. "Social Work and Speciesism." *Social Work* 45.1 (2000): 88–93.

Worldwatch Institute. "Worldwatch Institute: Vision for a Sustainable World." 26 Mar. 2009. *http://www.worldwatch.org/* (accessed 27 Mar. 2009).

Worsley, Anthony, and Grace Skrzypiec. "Teenage Vegetarianism:

Prevalence, Social and Cognitive Contexts." *Appetite* 30 (1998): 151–170.

Zey, Mary, and William Alex McIntosh. "Predicting Intent to Consume Beef: Normative Versus Attitudinal Influences." *Rural Sociology* 57.2 (1992): 250–265.

Zur, Ofer. "On Nuclear Attitudes and Psychic Numbing: Overview and Critique." *Contemporary Social Psychology* 14.2 (1990): 96–119.

Zwerdling, Daniel. "A View to a Kill." *Gourmet.* June 2007. *http://www.gourmet.com/magazine/2000s/2007/06/aviewtoakill* (accessed 26 Mar. 2009).

INDEX

heart diseases, 92
herbicides, 74
Herman, Judith, 139, 150
history, supporting naturalization, 108
Hitler, Adolf, 37, 143
hormones, 54, 60, 74, 86, 93, 144
horses, 130
Humane Methods of Slaughter Act, 54
Humane Society of the United States
    (HSUS), 41, 145
Human Rights Watch, 78
humans. *See also* health issues; slaughter
    workers
  aversion to killing, 34–35
  empathy and, 140
  food chain position and carnism
      justification, 108
  sentience studies and infants, 56, 57
  as victims of carnism, 74
Huxley, Aldous, 73

ideational disgust, 126, 131
identification, 126
ideologies
  defined, 30
  invisible, 28–32, 71–72
  justification of, 96–98, 105–107
  legitimization of, 103
  violent, 32–33, 71, 88, 93, 96, 112
impregnation, artificial, 47, 60–61
India, 85
inedible *vs.* edible classifications,
    14–16, 122–123, 129–132
infants, and sentience, 56, 57
inspections, 75–79
integration, 141
invisibility
  as defense mechanism, 21
  ideologies supported by, 28–32, 35,
      40–41, 67, 71–72
  literal *vs.* symbolic, 93
  weakening of, 146

Journal of Food Protection, 77
Jungle, The (Sinclair), 75–76
justifications, 96–97, 105–112

Kaplan, Helmut, 135
killing, human aversion to, 34–35
knowing without knowing, 71

Lama, Eddie, 143
language, 47–48, 118
LA Times, 59
legislation and legal system
  food libel laws, 91
  meat industry influence on, 89–90
  protecting animal enterprises, 41
  regulating quality control, 75–79
  regulating slaughter, 54
  status of animals, 103, 118
legitimization, 102–105
Lifton, Robert Jay, 87, 141
Little, Ellen, 136
live chilling, 66
lobbyists, 89–90
lobsters, 57, 64

mad cow disease, 67, 91
manure
  contamination from, 74–75, 77,
      78, 93
  environmental issues due to, 74,
      87, 144
Maple Leaf Foods, 47
Marshall, S. L. A., 34, 35
masculinity, 110
mastitis, 61
Matrix, The (film), 115–116, 134
McCartney, Sir Paul, 71, 145
McDonald's, 47
McKown, Delos B., 23
Meat Inspection Act, 75, 76
meatocracy, 91
meatpacking. *See* slaughterhouses and
    meatpacking

TO OUR READERS

Conari Press, an imprint of Red Wheel/Weiser, publishes books on topics ranging from spirituality, personal growth, and relationships to women's issues, parenting, and social issues. Our mission is to publish quality books that will make a difference in people's lives—how we feel about ourselves and how we relate to one another. We value integrity, compassion, and receptivity, both in the books we publish and in the way we do business.

Our readers are our most important resource, and we value your input, suggestions, and ideas about what you would like to see published. Please feel free to contact us, to request our latest book catalog, or to be added to our mailing list.

Conari Press
An imprint of Red Wheel/Weiser, LLC
500 Third Street, Suite 230
San Francisco, CA 94107
www.redwheelweiser.com